Reflex epilepsies

Reflex epilepsies

Progress in understanding

Editors:
Peter Wolf
Yushi Inoue
Benjamin Zifkin

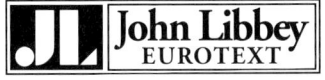

ISBN: 2-7420-0540-4
Current problems in epilepsy series: vol. 19
ISSN: 0950-4591

Éditions John Libbey Eurotext
127, avenue de la République, 92120 Montrouge, France
Tél. : 01 46 73 06 60
Editor : Maud Thévenin
Site internet : http://www.john-libbey-eurotext.fr

John Libbey Eurotext
42-46 High Street
Esher, Surrey
KT10 9KY
United Kingdom

© 2004, John Libbey Eurotext

Il est interdit de reproduire intégralement ou partiellement le présent ouvrage sans autorisation de l'éditeur ou du Centre Français d'Exploitation du Droit de Copie, 20, rue des Grands-Augustins, 75006 Paris.

List of Contributors

Andermann F., Department of Neurology and Neurosurgery, Montreal Neurological Institute and Hospital, McGill University, Montreal, Canada.

Ariki M., Department of Pediatrics, Gifu Prefectural Gifu Hospital, 4-6-1 Noishiki Gifu 500-8717, Japan.

Batini C., CNRS. Institut de Neurobiologie Alfred-Fessard, Gif-sur-Yvette, France and Université Pierre-et-Marie-Curie, CNRS UMR 7091, Paris, France.

Binnie C.D., Department of Clinical Neurophysiology, King's College Hospital, Denmark Hill, London SE5 9RS, United Kingdom.

Biraben A., Service de Neurologie, CHU Pontchaillou, rue Henri-Le-Guilloux, 35033 Rennes Cedex, France.

Braga N.I.O., Department of Neurology, Escola Paulista de Medicina, Universidade Federal de São Paulo, Rua Pedro de Toledo, 650, 04039-002. São Paulo, São Paulo, Brazil.

Carrete H., Department of Neurology, Escola Paulista de Medicina, Universidade Federal de São Paulo, Rua Pedro de Toledo, 650, 04039-002. São Paulo, São Paulo, Brazil.

Doury E., Service de Neurologie, CHU Pontchaillou, rue Henri-Le-Guilloux, 35033 Rennes Cedex, France.

Dubeau F., Department of Neurology and Neurosurgery, Montreal Neurological Institute and Hospital, McGill University, Montreal, Canada.

Fritsch B., The Interdisciplinary Epilepsy Center, Department of Neurology, Philipps-University Marburg, Germany.

Fujiwara S., Filtec Inc., 1214-1-614 Kunugida-cho Hatiouji, Tokyo 193-0942, Japan.

Garzon E., Department of Neurology, Escola Paulista de Medicina, Universidade Federal de São Paulo, Rua Pedro de Toledo, 650, 04039-002. São Paulo, São Paulo, Brazil.

Halasz P., National Institute of Psychiatry and Neurology, Budapest, Hungary.

Hattori S., Department of Pediatrics, Gifu Prefectural Gifu Hospital, 4-6-1 Noishiki Gifu 500-8717, Japan.

Inoue Y., National Epilepsy Center, Shizuoka Institute of Epilepsy and Neurological Disorders, Urushiyama 886, Shizuoka 420-8688, Japan.

Jimenez A.P., Department of Pediatrics, Hospital del Niño Jesus, Madrid, Spain.

Koepp M.J., Department of Clinical and Experimental Epilepsy, Institute of Neurology, National Hospital for Neurology, Queen Square, London WC1N 3BG, United Kingdom.

Matsuo N., Department of Pediatrics, Gifu Prefectural Gifu Hospital, 4-6-1 Noishiki Gifu 500-8717, Japan.

Mayer T., Saxion Epilepsy, Centre Kleinwachau, Radeberg, Germany.

Naquet R., CNRS. Institut de Neurobiologie Alfred-Fessard, Gif-sur-Yvette, France and Université Pierre-et-Marie-Curie, CNRS UMR 7091, Paris, France.

Noppeney U., Wellcome Department of Cognitive Neurology, Institute of Neurology, Institute of Neurology, National Hospital for Neurology, Queen Square, London WC1N 3BG, United Kingdom.

Palmini A., Porto Alegre Epilepsy Surgery Program, Hospital São Lucas, Pontificia Universidade Católica do Rio Grande do Sul (PUCRS), Porto Alegre, Brazil.

Plouin P., Hopital Necker Enfants malades, 149 rue de Sèvres, 75015 Paris, France.

Price C., Wellcome Department of Cognitive Neurology, Institute of Neurology, National Hospital for Neurology, Queen Square, London WC1N 3BG, United Kingdom.

Rosenow F., The Interdisciplinary Epilepsy Center, Department of Neurology, Philipps-University Marburg, Germany.

Sakamoto A.C., Department of Neurology, Escola Paulista de Medicina, Universidade Federal de São Paulo, Rua Pedro de Toledo, 650, 04039-002. São Paulo, São Paulo, Brazil.

Salek-Haddadi A., Department of Clinical and Experimental Epilepsy, Institute of Neurology, National Hospital for Neurology, Queen Square, London WC1N 3BG, United Kingdom.

Satishchandra P., Department of Neurology, National Institute of Mental Health & Neuro Sciences (NIMHANS), Bangalore, 560 029, India.

Sato T., Faculty of Textile Science, Kyoto Institute of Technology, Goshokaido-cho, Matsugasaki, Sakyo-ku, Kyoto 606-8585, Japan.

Scarabin J.M., Service de Neurologie, CHU Pontchaillou, rue Henri-Le-Guilloux, 35033 Rennes Cedex, France.

Schaeffer I., Austin and Repatriation Medical Center, University of Melbourne, Australia.

Schöndienst M., Klinik Mara I, Epilepsy Centre Bethel, Marawez 21, D-33617, Bielefeld.

Shankar S.K., Department of Neuropathology, National Institute of Mental Health & Neuro Sciences (NIMHANS), Bangalore, 560 029, India.

Skaff R., Department of Neurology, Escola Paulista de Medicina, Universidade Federal de São Paulo, Rua Pedro de Toledo, 650, 04039-002. São Paulo, São Paulo, Brazil.

Takahashi Y., National Epilepsy Center, Shizuoka Institute of Epilepsy and Neurological Disorders, Urushiyama 886, Shizuoka 420-8688, Japan.

Ullal G.R., Department of Psychology, Mcmaster University, Main Street West, Hamilton-Ontario, Canada 485 4K1.

Vigevano F., Ospedale Bambino Gesù, Piazza S. Onofrio 4, I 00165 Roma.

Wieser H.G., Abteilung für Epileptologie & Elektroenzephalographie, Neurologische Klinik, Universitätsspital, CH – 8091, Zürich.

Wolf P., Danish Epilepsy Centre Dianalund, Kolonivej 1, DK – 4293 Dianalund, Denmark.

Yacubian E.M.T., Department of Neurology, Escola Paulista de Medicina, Universidade Federal de São Paulo, Rua Pedro de Toledo, 650, 04039-002. São Paulo, São Paulo, Brazil.

Zifkin, B.G., Faculté de Médecine, Université de Montréal, Hôpital du Sacré-Cœur de Montréal; and Epilepsy Clinic, Montreal Neurological Hospital and Institute, Montreal, Quebec, Canada.

Foreword

Two valuable books on reflex seizures and reflex epilepsies have appeared in recent years, one edited by Beaumanoir, Gastaut and Naquet in 1989, and another by Zifkin, F. Andermann, Beaumanoir and Rowan in 1998. Now several years later, we have a new book on the same topic. The appearance of three books in this relatively short interval may reflect the active interest of epileptologists in reflex seizures. Much of this has been fuelled by the enormous advances in magnetic resonance imaging of morphology and function, in positron emission tomography of cognitive processing and in neurogenetics. But more importantly, the reflex seizures and epilepsies have attracted the attention of epileptologists because they can provide an important clue to the understanding of epileptogenesis. We have seen some progress also in this respect. The title of this new book *Reflex Epilepsies – Progress in Understanding* therefore has a double meaning: a) that the book reports progress in the understanding of reflex epilepsies, and b) that the book describes how the study of reflex seizures helps us to better understand epilepsy itself.

Distinguished epileptologists from around the world gathered in June 2001 at the 12th International Bethel-Cleveland Epilepsy Symposium, held in Bielefeld, Germany, to discuss and bring up to date our knowledge of the reflex epilepsies. The symposium covered almost all the modalities of reflex epilepsies: from photosensitivity in its clinical, experimental and therapeutic aspects, thermosensitive and eating modalities, induction by sensory stimuli and movement in different age groups, and cognitive and emotional aspects including triggering by music. Not only the variety of triggering factors, but also the mechanisms of reflex epileptogenesis were discussed in depth, as were their clinical manifestations. There was also description of novel reflex seizures such as perioral reflex myoclonia seen in *Juvenile Myoclonic Epilepsy*. Advances in functional imaging and neuropathology open a new era of understanding of the basic mechanisms of reflex epilepsy. These various aspects of discussion provided ideas for further consideration, especially for our nosological understanding of the epilepsies. It was interesting that some authors advanced, but in different ways, the idea that hyperexcitable regional or functional networks are involved in causing reflex seizures in patients with a "generalized epilepsy".

We thank the many individuals that have worked on this project, in particular our worldwide contributors and the local organizers of the Epilepsiezentrum Bethel. We are grateful for the help and support of the Bethel Foundation which allowed us to hold this symposium. We thank our publisher, John Libbey, and his staff for their advice and skill.

The editors

References

- Beaumanoir A, Gastaut H, Naquet R (eds). *Reflex seizures and reflex epilepsies*. Genève: Editions Médecine & Hygiène, 1989.
- Zifkin BG, Andermann F, Beaumanoir A, Rowan AJ (eds). *Reflex epilepsies and reflex seizures. Advances in Neurology Vol. 75*. Philadelphia: Lippincott-Raven, 1998.

Contents

Foreword
   P. Wolf, Y. Inoue, B. Zifkin VII

Introduction: contributions to the understanding of reflex epilepsies, and the reflex epilepsies contributions to the understanding of epilepsy
   P. Wolf... 1

Evidence of reflex epilepsy on functional systems in the brain and "generalised" epilepsy
   C.D. Binnie... 7

Varieties of photosensitivity in man ("plain" and progressive myoclonus epilepsies), in baboon and fowl
   R. Naquet, C. Batini 15

Prevention of photosensitive seizures by optical filters
   Y. Takahashi, S. Fujiwara, N. Matsuo, S. Hattori, M. Ariki, T. Sato 27

Praxis induction and thinking induction: one or two mechanisms? A controversy
   Y. Inoue, B. Zifkin.. 41

Perioral reflex myoclonias in reading epilepsy and juvenile myoclonic epilepsy
   T. Mayer, P. Wolf... 57

Fuctional imaging in reading epilepsy
   M.J. Koepp, U. Noppeney, A. Salek-Haddadi, C. Brice 71

Musicogenic seizures and findings on the anatomy of musical perception
   H.G. Wieser 79

Emotional seizure precipitation and psychogenic epileptic seizures
   M. Schöndienst 93

Trigger mechanisms in hot-water epilepsy
    P. Satishchandra, G.R. Ullal, S.K. Shankar.. 105

Reflex epileptic seizures in infancy
    P. Plouin, F. Vigevano... 115

Seizures induced by eating in a family
    E.M. Yacubian, R. Skaff, E. Garzon, N.I.O. Braga, A.C. Sakamoto,
    H. Carrete... 123

Motor reflex epilepsy induced by touch and movement
    A. Biraben, E. Doury, J.M. Scarabin 135

Malformations of cortical development as a cause of reflex seizures: neurobiological insights
    A. Palmini, P. Halász, I. Schaeffer, Y. Takahashi, A. Perez Jimenez,
    F. Dubeau, F. Andermann, F. Rosenow, B. Fritsch... 143

Introduction: contributions to the understanding of reflex epilepsies, and the reflex epilepsies' contributions to the understanding of epilepsy

P. Wolf

Danish Epilepsy Centre Dianalund, Dianalund, Denmark

One of the seeming paradoxes of the epilepsies is that, if an individual suffers from epilepsy, seizures do not occur all the time but only at intervals. Patients who seize every day are the exception, and in the majority of cases, seizures are relatively rare. This is one of the clearest indicators, in the natural history of epilepsy, that ictogenesis (*i.e.* the generation of seizures) in established epilepsy is by no means a one-dimensional process. There is probably a multitude of factors, synergistic and antagonistic, facilitating and counteracting the occurrence of seizures. Some of these we seem to know but there may be many others that still await discovery. The better we come to know these factors, the better we will be able to intervene and improve our therapy. But, beyond this practical purpose, the elucidation of these complex interactions will also improve our theoretical understanding of the basic mechanisms of epilepsy.

The so-called reflex epilepsies, a heterogeneous group of conditions where seizures are triggered, immediately or with short delays, by sensory or cognitive precipitating mechanisms, are a fascinating field of epileptology where we can gain most interesting insights, both qualitative and quantitative, into the generation of seizures.

Dr. Colin Binnie, who has devoted much of his work to photosensitivity (PhS), sets out with a discussion of ictogenesis in reflex epilepsy, using the example of PhS. In spite of the well-known affinity of PhS to the idiopathic generalised epilepsies (IGEs) (Wolf & Gooßes, 1986), various local actions can be demonstrated. Does this mean that the assumed relation of PhS to IGE is erroneous? This is not what follows, according to Binnie. He rather argues that something may be wrong with the concept of "generalised" epilepsies, and that it is in need of reconsideration. I couldn't agree more (Blume & Wolf, 1997; Wolf, 2003).

Is PhS, this best known of all reflex epileptic phenomena, as homogeneous at all as many seem to believe; a clear example of "generalised" epilepsy (if we still accept this concept for a moment), with a natural animal model attached to it, *i.e.* the photosensitive Senegalese baboon? *Dr. Robert Naquet*, the leading expert on photosensitive animals, together with his co-worker, *Dr. Cesira Batini*, presents an enlightening view of the variability of responses to intermittent light stimuli. Even in man, PhS is not homogeneous. "Plain" PhS differs from the PhS in progressive myoclonus epilepsies, but even plain PhS includes a variety of different responses. Variability also exists within the photosensitivities of the Senegalese baboon, and the Fayoumi chicken. The role of the brainstem is very clear in the latter – could it also exist in the higher species? The "magic" flicker frequency is the same in man and chicken but different in the ape. What could be the reason for this phylogenetic anomaly? This chapter leaves us with much food for thought.

One of the promises of the study of reflex mechanisms in ictogenesis is the possibility of therapies that act directly upon the trigger mechanisms, protecting the brain against their action (sensory protection, Wolf & Okujava, 1999). In PhS, the attenuation of the light stimulus is an obvious possibility that has been successfully applied (Harding & Jeavons, 1994). Several attempts have been made to refine this approach *e.g.* using polarised glasses (Vuong & Wolf, 1995) and blue lenses (Capovilla *et al.*, 1997). *Dr. Yukitoshi Takahashi* and his colleagues present the results of their investigations based on the famous POKEMON incident where hundreds of Japanese television watchers simultaneously had seizures precipitated by an intense visual stimulus in a TV programme – for many of them with unknown PhS the first seizure in life. They conclude that the suppression of long-wave red components of the light by protective lenses can be expected to be most efficient.

Drs. Yushi Inoue and Benjamin Zifkin then enter into an argument about the question whether praxis induction and seizures provoked by thinking are in fact one and the same, or two different reflex epileptic mechanisms. This discussion, however, does not stop at this rather preliminary controversy but moves on to a much more analytic consideration of the various cognitive and ideational processes which doubtlessly are to some extent involved in both varieties. Functional imaging increasingly allows us to pinpoint the brain areas that are activated during these processes. Analogies can be drawn to primary reading epilepsy (Wolf, 1994) which bears so many structural similarities to precipitation by praxis or thinking, but also to Dr. Binnie's above-mentioned discussion of the local components in the generation of photosensitive seizures.

Dr. Thomas Mayer adds a report on his enlightening discovery that perioral reflex myoclonias (PORM), which are the hallmark of primary reading epilepsy, are also a frequent trait in juvenile myoclonic epilepsy where they have been overlooked for many decades. This finding of a functional and semiological link connecting the prototype of an idiopathic "generalised" epilepsy syndrome with an idiopathic localisation-related syndrome underlines what Dr. Binnie pointed out in his chapter: that, in the field of the idiopathic epilepsies, the dichotomy of generalised *versus* focal ictogenesis is bound to dissolve in consequence of an improved understanding of the complex functional-anatomical circuits at play, some more widespread and more symmetric than others.

Dr. *Matthias Koepp* and his colleagues in their contribution on functional imaging in Reading Epilepsy provide an exemplary demonstration of how this could happen.

But also in musicogenic epilepsy, a type of reflex seizures which belongs to the realm of focal, often symptomatic epilepsies, functional anatomical investigations may contribute to a much more detailed understanding of their ictogenesis, as appears from *Dr. Heinz-Gregor Wieser's* chapter on this particular elaborate trigger mechanism.

Whereas Dr. Wieser concentrates on the neurology of musical perception, it has often been observed that, in many patients with musicogenic seizures, the emotional component of musical perception seems to be an indispensable part of the precipitating mechanism; it has even been suggested that musicogenic seizures should really be considered an emotional type of seizure precipitation. Musicogenic epilepsy thus seems to provide a link to this kind of triggers which have probably received too little attention – perhaps because they are difficult to pinpoint and quantify. *Dr. Martin Schöndienst* in this volume has taken the difficult task to discuss the provocation of seizures by affect and emotion. His thoughtful paper makes us better understand that it is mostly due to methodological problems that this topic has not yet received due attention. Sensory and even some cognitive precipitating factors are much more easy to define, detect, and operationalise for study than affects. The latter have a more complex structure and are often much less apparent. Also, they may be active as both direct precipitators, and as facilitators of seizures, the latter aspect being easier to study. However, with adequate methods these trigger mechanisms become accessible, and may open alleys to therapy that are as effective as the protection against sensory or cognitive stimuli.

Two variants of reflex epilepsy that still pose many unresolved questions are those with seizures precipitated by hot water and by eating. Both have been most frequently described on the Indian subcontinent, and *Dr. P. Satishchandra* and his colleagues give us an authentic account of their findings with trigger mechanisms for hot water epilepsy including an experimental animal model. They seem to indicate that a genetic insufficiency of thermoregulation is an important factor, and that these are really seizures triggered by hyperthermia. Since, typically, they are only provoked by water being poured over the head, and this is not done every day, patients with provoked seizures only can be treated by intermittent clobazam.

An updated description of the infantile variant of hot water epilepsy is then included in the chapter by *Drs. Perrine Plouin* and *Federico Vigevano*. Here, the spontaneous termination of the specific sensitivity at the age of three could indicate that, again, thermoregulation is involved as it becomes more efficient with growth. Here, however, the seizures occur when the baby's bottom is lowered into the bath. These authors also draw our attention to a variety of reflex myoclonic seizures in infants which are provoked by unexpected noises but are quite different from the usual startle epilepsy. Among the other types they report, they find that the trigger mechanism is still unclarified in eating seizures.

Dr. Elza Marcia Yacubian and her colleagues contribute to our understanding of this particular condition by a short review, and a report of a new family with eating-induced seizures, the first outside Sri Lanka. They highlight that there seems to be two types of seizures provoked by eating, one temporolimbic where a genetic mechanism seems to be involved, the other suprasylvian with symptomatic etiologies. But there seem also to be patients with generalised epilepsies, and Dr. Yacubian's discussion leads, again, to questioning the traditional dichotomy of generalised *versus* focal.

Dr. Arnaud Biraben and his co-authors discuss a type of reflex seizures which are certainly focal, and probably always symptomatic, although it has not in all cases been possible to demonstrate a morphological lesion: the reflex seizures of the perisylvian region which are induced by movement and touch. The authors convincingly argue that these really are variants of one type, and their discussion includes considerations of the pathophysiological mechanisms involved.

If it is true that the last-mentioned type is mostly due to cortical malformations, and pathophysiological explanations for that are not too difficult to find, *Dr. André Palmini* in the last chapter wonders why this pathology is not much more inclined to produce reflex seizures. For his contribution, he kindly has taken it on himself to collect nine cases with proven cortical malformations and reflex seizures from colleagues of seven different centres who became his co-authors. Interestingly, the reflex epilepsies observed are quite different and do not all belong, as could theoretically have been expected, to the type where the epileptic response is immediate, and anatomically directly related to the afferent stimulus. In the cases where it is, however, the seizure semiology reflects the anatomical location of the malformation.

A recurrent issue in the contributions to this book is the growing awareness that our traditional concept of generalised epileptic conditions as opposed to focal, mostly symptomatic epilepsies, does not any more reflect our understanding of ictogenesis. The study of well-defined trigger mechanisms leads up again and again to concepts of central nervous subsystems acting as pathological networks or circuits that interact to generate seizures. At least as far as reflex epilepsies are concerned, the "generalised" types seem to be system epilepsies with a roughly symmetrical expression and the localisation-related types, system epilepsies with a much more asymmetric expression. It is therefore thought-provoking that in a syndrome like juvenile myoclonic epilepsy, now generally considered as the core syndrome of idiopathic "generalised" epilepsies, reflex epileptic traits are so widespread that very few if any patients with this condition do not present at least one of them. The most important contribution to the study of reflex epilepsies in recent years seems thus to have been to our nosological understanding of the epilepsies.

References

1. Blume WT, Wolf P. Introduction to the Epilepsies. In: Engel J Jr, Pedley TA, eds. *Epilepsy. A Comprehensive Textbook*. Philadelphia & New York: Lippincott-Raven, 1997: 765-72.
2. Capovilla G, Mussini P, Paladin F, Romeo A, Veggiotti PA, Sgrò V, Canger R. Utilizzo di lenti sperimentali blu nel controllo della fotosensibilità. *Boll Lega It Epil* 1997; 98: 5-9.
3. Harding GFA, Jeavons PM. *Photosensitive Epilepsy. New Edition*. London: Mac Keith, 1994.
4. Vuong TA, Wolf P. Polarisierte Brillengläser als Anfallsschutz bei Fotosensibilität. *Epilepsie-Blätter* 1995; 8 (suppl. 1): 30.
5. Wolf P. Of Cabbages and Kings: Some Considerations on Classifications, Diagnostic Schemes, Semiology, and Concepts. *Epilepsia* 2003; 44: 1-4.
6. Wolf P, Gooßes R. Relation of photosensitivity to epileptic syndromes. *J Neurol Neurosurg Psychiat* 1986; 49: 1386-91.
7. Wolf P, Okujava N. Possibilities of nonpharmacological conservative treatment of epilepsy. *Seizure* 1999; 8: 45-52.

Evidence of reflex epilepsy on functional systems in the brain and "generalised" epilepsy

C.D. Binnie

King's College, London, UK

■ Introduction

The 1981 and 1989 ILAE classifications of seizures and of epilepsy syndromes (Commission on Classification and Terminology of ILEA, 1981; 1989) rely heavily on maintaining a distinction between primarily generalised, focal, and secondarily generalised epileptogenesis. These concepts have proved valuable as aids to teaching and communication, have promoted a greater awareness of ictal semiology and of different epilepsy syndromes, and have facilitated the current rapid developments in the genetics of epilepsy. Nevertheless, the pathophysiological assumptions on which they are based are suspect (Binnie, 1994). This appears to underlie the thinking of an ILAE task force that has recently recommended in effect the abandonment of attempts at such rigorous classification (Engel, 2001). One may now be pushing at an open door by discussing this matter at all, but if classification in epilepsy has been reconsidered, some credit may be claimed for evidence from observations on reflex epilepsies.

The critique of the generalised/focal dichotomy centres on evidence of local structural or functional abnormality, and particularly epileptogenesis, in epilepsies and seizures considered as "primarily" generalised. Evidence may be drawn from many sources.

1. Structural abnormalities in the form of focal cortical dysgenesis are reported in idiopathic generalised epilepsy (IGE) (Meencke & Janz, 1984; Woermann *et al.*, 1999).

2. Local functional abnormalities may be directly demonstrable by neuroimaging, for instance in the mesial frontal region, in IGE (Koepp & Duncan, 2000).

3. Postulated diffuse cortical hyperexcitability in IGE is not necessarily uniform, as evidenced by both spontaneous and reflex epileptogenesis:

- *EEG and seizure semiology may indicate asymmetric or focal cortical activation.*
- EEG:
  Focal interictal discharges occur in IGE, e.g. 34% in JME (Panayiotopoulos et al., 1991).
  There is a high prevalence of asymmetrical discharge onsets (32%) & foci (39%) in IGE (Binnie, 1996).
- Seizure semiology:
  Versive or rotatory seizures occur in JME.
  Otherwise typical absences may involve version.
  Careful video analysis often shows a craniocaudal march in absences (Stefan, 1981).

- *Reflex epileptogenesis:*
- Specific activities (sensory, motor or cognitive) can selectively activate epileptogenesis in specific cortical regions, with appropriate electrographic and clinical sequelae.
- Specific regions may be more susceptible to such activation than homologous areas in the opposite hemisphere.

Only the evidence from reflex epileptogenesis falls within the scope of the present review.

Focal Reflex Epileptogenesis in IGE: Photosensitivity

The diffuse cortical hyperexcitability postulated in IGE, as assessed by responses to stimuli, is not necessarily uniform. The best evidence comes from studies of photosensitivity. Photosensitivity, elicited by flicker (IPS), and particularly pattern, has been extensively studied, and since the pioneering work of Hubel and Wiesel (1968), the cellular physiological concomitants of pattern vision have been well documented. Hence, from the physical characteristics determining the epileptogenicity of patterns, inferences may be drawn concerning the pathophysiology of epileptogenesis (e.g. Wilkins et al., 1980).

Reflex Epileptogenesis in P. papio

The Senegalese baboon shows a genetic or pharmacologically induced generalised epilepsy not associated with any structural abnormality. Exposure to flicker over some minutes produces progressively recruiting generalised EEG discharges and myoclonus.

Discharges are initiated in frontocentral cortex, before other cortical or subcortical structures (Fischer-Williams et al., 1968), and generalisation is secondary. In frontal cortex, single unit bursts are synchronous with spike-wave activity, but in the occipital region they are time-locked to the flashes as in the normal brain (Menini et al., 1981). Repeated flashes elicit progressively recruiting giant evoked potentials in the frontal, but not the visual cortex. Frontocentral epileptogenesis is abolished by ablation of occipital cortex (Lanoir & Dimov, 1971). Callosotomy desynchronises the discharges between hemispheres (Naquet et al., 1972) and, after callosotomy, hemifield stimulation produces only contralateral discharges (Fukuda et al., 1989), therefore corticocortical rather than thalamocortical pathways are involved.

Thus P. papio exhibits a stimulus-induced partial epilepsy arising in the frontal cortex, with secondary generalisation. The afferent signals are relayed via the visual cortex by unilateral, probably corticocortical pathways. Each frontal lobe is independently capable of epileptogenesis, and bilateral synchrony depends on transcallosal connections. This then is a typical generalised epilepsy, either idiopathic or induced by diffuse cerebral exposure to a convulsive agent, in which physiological dissection demonstrates focal epileptogenesis in each frontal lobe.

Mechanisms of Photosensitivity in Man

Human photosensitivity has some features in common with that of P. papio. It is ordinarily genetically determined, but may be induced by pharmacological means (notably abrupt withdrawal of anticonvulsant agents). The epilepsy syndrome is typically idiopathic generalised. However, the pathophysiology of photosensitivity is significantly different. Discharges are initiated in parieto-occipital cortex; recruitment is much more rapid than in P. papio, but again the generalisation is secondary. Epileptogenesis depends on stimulus characteristics that determine patterns of neuronal activity in visual cortex, namely:

1. level of activity within a specific neuronal population;
2. volume of cortex activated in either hemisphere;
3. propagation from the parieto-occipital area;
4. synchronisation of activity by spatiotemporal characteristics of stimulus.

(1) to (3) of the above are relevant to the current topic of classification.

Unless otherwise stated, these conclusions follow chiefly from the work of Wilkins et al. (1980) on pattern sensitivity:

1. Stimulus characteristics that determine discharge occurrence are those which determine activity levels of parieto-occipital cortical neurones in experimental animals. Epileptogenicity is maximised by:

- A spatial frequency of 2-4 cycles/degree.

- Continuous line contours within the pattern: stripes are more effective than rectangles, and these are more effective than checkerboards.

- Binocular fusion: monocular flicker stimulation reduces epileptogenicity to a degree roughly equivalent to that of reducing stimulus intensity by 90%. The epileptogenicity of binocular pattern stimuli that are effective under conditions of fusion (i.e. when identical patterns are exposed to each eye) is abolished or much reduced if the pattern presented to one eye is rotated through 20° with respect to the other, preventing fusion.

2. Stimuli close to threshold elicit discharges confined to the posterior regions:

- Marginally supraliminal hemifield pattern stimulation elicits discharges over the contralateral posterior quadrant (Wilkins et al., 1981).

- Discharges elicited by either IPS or pattern may remain confined posteriorly for seconds before generalising, if the stimulus is marginally supraliminal or if generalisation is suppressed by valproate.
- Subliminal IPS at 8 Hz may elicit abnormal steady state VEPs, which persist even after generalised discharges are abolished by valproate (Harding et al., 1978).

3. Discharges arise when the pattern projects to a critical cortical area, within each hemisphere separately:

- Discharge probability increases with the area of cortical projection of the pattern. Peripheral and central stimuli (e.g. annuli and discs) projecting to different areas of cortex are of equivalent epileptogenicity after correction for the cortical magnification factor (i.e. a small pattern disc in central vision may be as effective as a large annulus at the periphery).
- Spatial summation between effects of discrete patterned stimuli occurs within each visual field independently, but not between fields. That is, epileptogenesis occurs independently in each hemisphere without summation of effects through the corpus callosum.
- Threshold pattern area may differ between hemispheres (Wilkins et al., 1981).
- When generalised discharges have been selectively suppressed by sodium valproate, the probability of posterior discharges is reduced, yet threshold pattern size remains unchanged (Darby et al., 1985).

Binocularly innervated contour-detecting complex cells showing orientation specificity are apparently confined to the visual cortex in primates. Hence the visual cortex plays a crucial role in epileptogenesis in the photosensitive human. Other evidence cited above indicates that it is not only crucial but is indeed the site in which recognisable epileptiform discharges first appear:

- Marginally supraliminal stimuli elicit posterior discharges; these may then be seen to generalise.
- Hemifield pattern stimulation activates the contralateral posterior quadrant.
- Threshold pattern size is asymmetrical in 50% of patients – as commonly in IGE as in other epilepsies.
- Responses to IPS are larger on the side with lower threshold to pattern.
- Subliminal 8 Hz flicker elicits occipital spikes, resistant to valproate.

In summary, epileptogenesis due to photosensitivity is initiated in parieto-occipital area; human photosensitivity, like that in P. papio is a model of partial epilepsy with secondary generalisation.

A feature of particular interest of the photosensitivity model is that apart from a liability to excessive, hypersynchronous discharge, the visual system appears to be functionally normal, as assessed by acuity, stereopsis and colour vision. Specifically, perception of gratings at threshold contrast is normal (Soso et al., 1980; Wilkins, 1995); a function that should be impaired if there were a failure of inhibitory mechanisms. This may suggest that, even if inhibitory failure can contribute to epileptogenesis, it is not a necessary cause. The only evidence of visual cortical abnormality is not directly related to epileptogenesis but to pattern reversal visual evoked potentials; these show a lack of luminance contrast gain control at low spatial frequencies (Porchiatti et al., 2000). Curiously, this is seen only at temporal frequencies lower than those that are most usually epileptogenic, and its relevance to mechanisms of photosensitivity is therefore uncertain. Probably a major factor in photosensitivity, and the predominance of this over all other forms of reflex epilepsy, is simply that the visual system provides a greater afferent input to the brain than does any other sensory modality.

Photosensitivity and Classification

The physiological studies cited above indicate that both in P. papio and Man, photogenic epileptogenesis arises in a circumscribed area of cortex and that generalisation of discharges is secondary. This is supported by clinical evidence.

Photosensitivity is strongly associated with idiopathic generalised epilepsy and there is a general perception that myoclonus, absences and tonic-clonic seizures are the typical clinical manifestations. Partial seizures, by contrast, are variously reported to be very rare (2.5% of photosensitive patients, Jeavons & Harding, 1975), or quite uncommon but occasionally seen as a specific syndrome (17% of patients overall, Guerrini et al., 1998). Perhaps for these reasons, when a photosensitive patient reports generalised seizures it may seem unnecessary to question them closely about the details. The present author has been as guilty as any of this omission.

It is striking that patients often describe tonic-clonic seizures occurring some minutes after exposure to a potentially epileptogenic stimulus has ended and it is all too easy to dismiss this as fortuitous. However, careful questioning typically elicits a different account. The patient became unwell whilst exposed to the stimulus, withdrew from the situation, turned off the television for example, and possibly went to seek help, may have become confused, and after a gradual evolution over several minutes through simple and complex partial semiology suffered a secondarily generalised convulsion. This is supported by a phenomenon that is uncommon and poorly documented but appears to be familiar to many workers in EEG laboratories, namely the occurrence of sharply focal unilateral occipital discharges, induced by IPS, that continue after stimulation and relentlessly evolve often over several minutes, culminating in a generalised seizure.

Indeed it appears that in a majority, some 65%, of patients with seizures induced by environmental visual stimuli, these have on occasion been of simple partial onset, typically but not invariably with visual symptoms but often with lateralising features (Hennessy & Binnie, 2000). Such seizures commonly occur in patients with idiopathic generalised epilepsy. They do not constitute a reason to revise the diagnosis or to exhibit drugs more suitable for partial epilepsies; however, they should encourage reconsideration of the concept of IGE.

It was noted above that hemifield pattern stimulation may elicit focal discharges over the contralateral posterior quadrant and that the threshold pattern size may be grossly asymmetrical, indeed pattern sensitivity may be apparently unilateral. IPS-induced discharges, even if rapidly generalising, appear first over the hemisphere with the lower pattern threshold (Binnie *et al.*, 1981; Wilkins *et al.*, 1981). Such asymmetry is found in some 50% of patients but is equally common in photosensitive subjects with idiopathic generalised, symptomatic partial, and symptomatic/cryptogenic generalised epilepsies. Thus it indicates an asymmetry of cortical hyperexcitability that may itself be bilateral, and is unrelated to gross pathology.

■ Evidence from Other Reflex Epilepsies

Triggering of seizures by simple, unstructured stimuli in sensory modalities other than vision is rare, if one excludes those in which startle is a major factor. Somatosensory induced seizures are mostly seen in patients with unilateral structural abnormalities in the somatosensory area and the seizures are appropriately lateralised and presumably reflect cortical hyperexcitability in the sensory cortex (Forster, 1969; Goldie & Green, 1959). Movement-induced seizures may have a similar mechanism due to proprioceptive feedback. Interestingly, Goldie and Green (1959) were able to elicit seizures and EEG discharge by hypnotic suggestion of the trigger stimulus, suggesting a role for perceptual rather than simple sensory mechanisms.

In reflex epilepsies with complex cognitive triggers the stimulus or psychological activity that elicits attacks may be highly specific, a particular visual image, voice, musical work, type of text or mental activity. It might be expected that these would in turn activate highly specific neural circuits, whether localised in accordance with classical neuropsychology or more widely distributed. Hyperexcitability in such circuits would in turn appear more likely to occur in partial epilepsies. However, with the exception of primary reading epilepsy this is not generally the case; cognitive triggering is mainly seen in idiopathic generalised epilepsy. Notably, in a substantial population of patients with epilepsy a battery of cognitive challenges elicited epileptiform activity in as many as 7.9%, of whom 95% had idiopathic generalised epilepsy (Matsuoka *et al.*, 2000).

■ Conclusion

It is clear that the postulated diffuse cortical hyperexcitability in IGE is not necessarily uniform, and that specific activities (sensory, motor or cognitive) can selectively activate specific localised regions of a diffusely hyperexcitable cortex. Such activation can produce focal discharges or partial seizures, which may remain focal or generalise. In either case, these should not cause the diagnosis of IGE to be questioned, but show the distinction between partial and generalised epileptogenesis implicit in traditional classifications to be simplistic and in need of reconsideration.

References

1. Binnie CD. Epilepsy in adults: diagnostic EEG investigation. In: Kimura J, Shibasaki H, eds. *Recent Advances in Clinical Neurophysiology*. Amsterdam: Elsevier, 1996; 217-22.
2. Binnie CD, Wilkins AJ, De Korte RA. Interhemispheric differences in photosensitive epilepsy: II. intermittent photic stimulation. *Electroencephalogr Clin Neurophysiol* 1981; 52: 469-72.
3. Binnie CD. An electrophysiological view. In: Wolf P, ed. *Epileptic Seizures and Syndromes*. London: John Libbey, 1994; 270-1.
4. Commission on Classification and Terminology of the International League Against Epilepsy. Proposal for revised clinical and electroencephalographic classification of epileptic seizures. *Epilepsia* 1981; 22: 489-501.
5. Commission on Classification and Terminology of the International League Against Epilepsy. Proposal for revised classification of epilepsies and epileptic syndromes. *Epilepsia* 1989; 30: 389-99.
6. Darby CE, Park, DM, Smith, AT, Wilkins, AJ. Electroencephalographic characteristics of epileptic pattern sensitivity and their relation to the nature of pattern stimulation and the effect of sodium valproate. *Electroencephalogr Clin Neurophysiol* 1985; 63: 517.
7. Engel J. A proposed diagnostic scheme for people with epileptic seizures and epilepsy: Report of the ILAE task force on classification and terminology. *Epilepsia* 2001; 42: 796-803.
8. Fischer-Williams M, Ponset M, Riche D, Naquet R. Light-induced epilepsy in the baboon Papio papio: cortical and depth recordings. *Electroencephalogr Clin Neurophysiol* 1968; 25: 557-69.
9. Forster FM. Somatosensory evoked epilepsy. *Trans Am Neurol Assoc* 1969; 94: 268-9.
10. Fukuda H, Valin A, Menini C, Boscher C, de-la-Sayette V, Riche D, Kunimoto M, Wada JA, Naquet R. Effect of macular and peripheral retina coagulation on photosensitive epilepsy in the forebrain bisected baboon Papio papio. *Epilepsia* 1989; 30: 623-30.
11. Goldie L, Green JM. A study of the psychological factors in a case of reflex epilepsy. *Brain* 1959; 82: 502-24.
12. Guerrini R, Bonanni P, Parmeggiani L, Thomas P, Mattia D, Harvey AS, Duchowny MS. Induction of partial seizures by visual stimulation. *Adv Neurol* 1998; 75: 159-78.
13. Harding GFA, Herrick CE, Jeavons PM. A controlled study of the effect of sodium valproate on photosensitive epilepsy and its prognosis. *Epilepsia* 1978; 19: 555.
14. Hennessy MJ, Binnie CD. Photogenic partial seizures. *Epilepsia* 2000; 41: 59-64.
15. Hubel DH, Wiesel TN. Receptive fields and functional architecture of monkey striate cortex. *J Physiol* 1968; 195: 229-89.
16. Jeavons PM, Harding GFA. Photosensitive epilepsy. London: Heinemann, 1975.
17. Koepp M, Duncan J. Positron emission tomography in idiopathic generalised epilepsy: imaging beyond structure. In: Schmidt D, ed. *Juvenile Myoclonic Epilepsy: the Janz Syndrome*. Petersfield: Rightson Biomedical Publications, 2000; 91-100.
18. Lanoir J, Dimov, S. Effets des foyers chroniques frontaux, temporaux et rolandiques chez le Papio papio photosensible. In: Usunoff G, ed. *Pathogenesis of Epilepsy*. Sofia: Bulgarian Academy of Sciences, 1971; 319-26.
19. Menini C, Stutzmann JM, Laurent H, Dimov S. Cortical unit discharges during photic stimulation in the Papio papio. Relationships with paroxysmal frontorolandic activity. *Electroencephalogr Clin Neurophysiol* 1981; 52: 42-9.
20. Matsuoka K, Takahashi T, Saoki M, *et al*. Neuropsychological EEG activation in patients with epilepsy. *Brain* 2000; 123: 318.
21. Meencke HJ, Janz D. Neuropathological findings in primary generalised epilepsy. *Epilepsia* 1984; 25: 8-21.

22. Naquet R, Menini C, Catier J. Photically induced epilepsy in Papio papio: the initiation of discharges and the role of frontal cortex and of the corpus callosum. In: Brazier MAB, Petsche H, eds. *Synchronization of the EEG in the Epilepsies*. Vienna: Springer Verlag, 1972; 347-67.
23. Panayiotopoulos CP, Tahan R, Obeid T. Juvenile myoclonic epilepsy: factors of error involved in the diagnosis and treatment. *Epilepsia* 1991; 32: 672-6.
24. Porchiatti V, Bonanni P, Fiorentini A, Guerrini R. Lack of cortical contrast gain control in human photosensitive epilepsy. *Nature Neurosci* 2000; 3: 259-63.
25. Soso MJ, Lettich E, Belgum JH. Case report: responses to stripe width changes and to complex gratings of patient with pattern-sensitive epilepsy. *Electroencephalogr Clin Neurophysiol* 1980; 48: 98-101.
26. Stefan H. Pseudospontanbewegungen bei Patienten mit Petit-mal-Anfällen. *Arch Psychiatrie Nervenkr* 1981; 229: 277-90.
27. Wilkins AJ, Binnie CD, Darby CE. Visually induced seizures. *Prog Neurobiol* 1980; 15: 85-117.
28. Wilkins AJ, Binnie CD, Kasteleijn-Nolst Trenité DGA, De Korte RA. Interhemispheric differences in photosensitivity. *Electroencephalogr Clin Neurophysiol* 1981; 52: 7.
29. Wilkins AJ. *Visual Stress*. Oxford: Oxford University Press, 1995.
30. Woermann FG, Free SL, Koepp MJ, et al. Abnormal cerebral structure in juvenile myoclonic epilepsy demonstrated with voxel-based analysis of MRI. *Brain* 1999; 122: 2101-7.

Varieties of photosensitivity in man ("plain" and progressive myoclonus epilepsies), in baboon and in fowl

R. Naquet, C. Batini

CNRS, Institut de Neurobiologie Alfred-Fessard, Gif-sur-Yvette, France and Université Pierre-et-Marie-Curie, CNRS UMR 7091, Paris, France

■ Introduction

In three species, Man (Cobb, 1947), Baboon Papio papio (Killam et al., 1966a) and Fayoumi chicken (Crawford, 1970), some subjects, who may or may not have presented epileptic seizures, show a particular response to intermittent light stimulation (ILS). This response, which has been well studied, has the characteristics of a paroxysmal response (PR), and the affected subjects are called "photosensitive". The PR may be only clinical (behavioural), only electroencephalographic (EEG) or both. Since it is induced by a sensory stimulus, it is classified among the "reflex epilepsies". Although the question of the definition is still open, we call "reflex" epilepsies those that need a sensory stimulus to precipitate seizures (Beaumanoir et al., 1989). This means that the subjects have a predisposition to epilepsy, but may not be aware of it unless exposed to the specific epileptogenic stimulus.

The predisposition of the subjects to present ILS-induced PR may be acquired, but more frequently is genetically determined or at least familial (in Man: Nekhorocheff, 1950; Doose et al., 1969; Doose & Gerken, 1973; in Papio papio: Balzamo et al., 1974; Naquet, 1975; in chicken: Crawford, 1970). The PR characteristics are different between species but vary also in the same species depending on the neurological disorder of the subject *(man)*, on the experimental lesion or transformation performed *(baboon and chicken)*, or on the pharmacologically induced modification *(the three species)*. The ILS-induced PRs of the three species are controlled in the same manner under treatment by anticonvulsant drugs, particularly by those enhancing the GABA efficacy (Naquet & Meldrum, 1985; Johnson et al., 1974; Johnson & Davis, 1883). In addition, in the baboon, the excitatory amino acid antagonists are also antiepileptic drugs (Chapman & Meldrum, 1993; Chapman, 1994).

We will describe at first, separately in each species, the characteristic expression of their excessive photosensitivity. We will then try, in the discussion, to analyse such data in view of identifying the circuits involved in the various types of ILS-induced PR.

The data presented will be voluntarily schematic. However, one should be aware that, particularly in man, more complex ILS-induced responses were found, particularly those secondary to the association of diverse aetiologies (Beaumanoir et al., 1989; Kasteleijn-Nolst Trenité, 1989; Kasteleijn-Nolst Trenité et al., 1994).

■ Clinical and EEG Symptoms

In Man (see: Gastaut, 1951; Bickford et al., 1952; Gastaut et al., 1958; Kooi et al., 1960; see also in Gastaut & Broughton, 1972; Klass & Fischer-Williams, 1975; Newmark & Penry, 1979; Naquet & Poncet-Ramade, 1982; Kasteleijn-Nolst Trenité, 1989; Kasteleijn-Nolst Trenité et al., 1994; Harding & Jeavons, 1994).

Clinical and EEG background of subjects presenting PR under ILS

Part of these subjects have no epileptic seizures, and some are considered as "entirely normal"; others are known to suffer from epilepsy, having spontaneously myoclonias, absences and/or *grand mal* seizures; another part are patients without epilepsy who are under treatment or intoxicated by substances diminishing the GABA cerebral level or enhancing the excitatory amino acid level.

The EEG may be normal at rest or may present paroxysmal discharges (PD) unilateral or bilateral in the occipital regions and/or in the frontorolandic (FR) regions, mostly bilateral.

EEG and clinical effects of ILS

The best ILS frequency to obtain PRs is called the *"magic frequency"* (Walter et al., 1948). *In man it is around 15 Hz.*

ILS particularly at this frequency may induce various types of symptoms belonging to the following syndromes. They generally reveal a "plain" photosensitivity.

1. Photo-Myoclonic response or Eyelid Myoclonias. These myoclonias follow the ILS frequency and enhance in amplitude progressively with ILS duration (Klass & Fischer-Williams, 1976; Naquet & Poncet-Ramade, 1982; Harding & Jeavons, 1994). They are associated to potentials recorded in the frontopolar region and have the same frequency and the same increasing amplitude of the myoclonia. These frontopolar recorded potentials are generally considered as muscle artefacts having no EEG origin (Gastaut, 1951; Bickford et al., 1952). However, some authors (Artieda & Obeso, 1993) claim that, in individual cases, superposed to artefacts there are frontorolandic paroxysmal responses (FRPRs) although no visible occipital PDs are detected. This photomyoclonic response is a rare phenomenon, found in old subjects, suffering from epilepsy or not. The myoclonias stop generally with the ILS cessation.

However, in some subjects they spread to the face, neck, and the all body and in the same time real PDs appears in the FR area (FRPDs). A typical *grand mal* may follow (Naquet & Poncet-Ramade, 1982; Beaumanoir et al., 1989).

2. Occipital PDs without clinical symptoms. These PDs are present in the occipital area where they do not follow the ILS frequency. They are often asymmetric, but they may also be bilateral and symmetric. They are found in photosensitive patients (although not in all of them). When they exist they are independent of the FRPDs (Lloyd-Smith & Henderson, 1951; Robertson, 1954; Gastaut et al., 1958; Panayotopoulos et al., 1972).

3. Clinical and EEG occipital seizures (Naquet et al., 1960; Beaumanoir et al., 1989). These ILS-induced EEG seizures do not follow the ILS frequency and persist after the end of ILS as an afterdischarge. They are generally unilateral, and they may be induced alternately in one or the other hemisphere of the same subject. They are found in people with and without epilepsy and, when they exist, the patient is generally photosensitive. Considered as a rare phenomenon in the early sixties, they are frequently observed at present in subjects playing video games (Badinand et al., 1998). They may:

- follow or not a burst of PDs in the frontorolandic area (FRPDs);
- stay localised in the occipital area and be accompanied clinically only by a transitory loss of vision in the visual field corresponding to the occipital cortex affected by PDs;
- spread to the anterior ipsilateral region, being then accompanied by progressive clinical symptoms corresponding to each new area of the cortex affected by PDs.

4. Frontorolandic PDs (FRPDs), or Photoconvulsive response (Gastaut, 1951; Bickford et al., 1952; Jeavons, 1969). These are made of spikes and waves and of polyspikes and waves appearing at the frequency of 3 Hz and therefore not following the ILS frequency. They have no clinical expression or they are associated with "generalised" myoclonias (each myoclonia corresponding to a spike or to the spike of a polyspike and wave). When the ILS induces polyspikes and the myoclonias become very intense, a typical *grand mal* seizure may follow. In patients affected by *absences*, these can be induced. The PDs may be the only symptom, the sign of the predisposition to photosensitive epilepsy. They are found more frequently in the adolescent females than in the male patients (Doose et al., 1969).

5. Frontorolandic visual evoked potentials (FRVEPs) and FRPDs in "Progressive Myoclonus Epilepsies" (and in some other neurodegenerative syndromes). FRVEPs are induced by single or double flashes and are generally not accompanied by clinical signs. Only in rare cases (Naquet, 1973) each double flash evokes partial myoclonias observed in the big toes. In these patients, however, short bursts of ILS-induced polyspikes and waves (FRPDs called giant PDs) are associated with "generalised" myoclonias.

In *Papio Papio* (Killam et al., 1966a, b, 1967; Fischer-Williams et al., 1968; Naquet & Meldrum, 1985; Menini & Naquet, 1986; Menini et al., 1994; Naquet & Valin, 1998).

Clinical and EEG background of subjects presenting PR under ILS

The animals affected are normal subjects at rest with or without exaggerated startle response. Very exceptionally they present spontaneous *grand mal* seizures.

The EEG at rest is normal or shows few isolated FRPD, independent of the startle response. PDs are never recorded in the occipital cortex.

EEG and clinical effects of ILS

The "magic frequency" is around 25 Hz. ILS, particularly at this frequency, induces four different kinds of signs of "plain" photosensitivity:

1. <u>Frontorolandic PDs</u>. Visual evoked potentials following the ILS frequency appear in FR areas, augment progressively in amplitude and finally become paroxysmal (FRPDs). When reaching a certain amplitude they become true FRPDs (also called giant PDs) which do not follow the ILS frequency. They are spikes or polyspikes and waves appearing at the frequency of 6 Hz. Eyelid myoclonias, if present, are, at the beginning, concomitant to the FRPDs and have therefore the ILS frequency; later on, they follow the modifications of the FRPDs. The eyelid myoclonias may: a) not spread, disappearing progressively before the FRPDs, or b) spread to the face and, more or less quickly, invade the whole body thus becoming true "generalised" myoclonias which may precipitate a seizure.

2. <u>Clinical and EEG FR seizures</u>. They generally follow a burst of ILS-induced FRPDs associated to "generalised" myoclonias. They are bilateral and synchronous and are particularly evident in the forelimbs. They are associated with a rhythmic PD on the EEG, localised bilaterally in the FR areas and outlasting the ILS arrest as an afterdischarge.

3. <u>Clinical and EEG *grand mal* seizures</u>. Typical *grand mal* seizure follow the "generalised" myoclonias associated to high amplitude ILS-induced FRPDs. The EEG at the beginning is characterised by a high frequency/low amplitude FR discharge. Rapidly with amplitude enhancement and slowing frequency, these discharges invade all the brain structures as in typical *grand mal* seizures. After injection of a substance diminishing the cerebral GABA level, the pattern may be different: the ILS-induced EEG seizure start bilaterally in the occipital lobe (Meldrum *et al.*, 1970).

4. <u>Highly photosensitive Papio papio</u>. Double flashes induce FRPDs but only when preceded by a burst of ILS at 25 Hz. Such facilitation to provoke FRPDs is also observed in normal animals injected with subliminal doses of allylglycine (Menini *et al.*, 1980).

Experimental modifications of EEG and clinical effects of ILS

Using different technologies it is possible to modify the ILS-induced PRs. Various examples of atypical *grand mal* seizures can be mentioned:

- The simple section of corpus callosum induces, under classical ILS, a discrete asynchrony between the two hemispheres of clinical and EEG *grand mal* discharges (Naquet et al., 1972) and, under unilateral ILS, a unilateral seizure (Fukuda et al., 1988).
- When the section of corpus callosum is associated a) to lesion of the temporal quadrant of the retina, ILS induces unilateral clinical and EEG seizures if directed only to the eye with lesioned retina (Fukuda et al., 1989); b) to unilateral FR lesions, ILS directed to both eyes induce unilateral clinical and EEG seizures in the intact hemisphere (Naquet & Wada, 1992).
- An appropriate unilateral (or bilateral) GABA injection in FR cortex block the EEG and clinical ILS-induced PDs (Brailowsky et al., 1989).

In Fowl (Crawford, 1970; Batini et al., 1996).

Clinical and EEG background of subjects presenting PR under ILS

The epileptic fowls (Fayoumi chicken or Fepi) seem to behave normally. Some of them may have presented myoclonias or generalised seizures, spontaneously or induced by a stimulus not clearly identified.

EEG consists of continuous Paroxysmal Slow Waves (PSW) and PDs.

EEG and clinical effects of ILS

The "magic frequency" is around 14 Hz. Clinically, the first sign is neck myoclonia, following the ILS frequency, quickly spreading to the whole body and usually inducing a generalised seizure recalling a *grand mal* fit. The seizure is followed by a short phase of stupor. Generalised seizures, but not neck myoclonia, outlast ILS (Crawford, 1970).

The first EEG sign is PSW and PDs blockage associated with desynchronisation of the rhythms that start soon after the beginning of ILS and persist during the myoclonia and the seizure and may be followed by a transitory depression (Guy et al., 1992). During ILS, and particularly at the beginning of the myoclonia, bursts of spikes having the ILS frequency and increasing in duration appears in the anterior tectum (Guy et al., 1993).

Experimental modifications of EEG and clinical effects of ILS

Birds are susceptible to embryonic manipulation which produce brain chimeras (Le Douarin, 1969; 1993; Le Douarin et al., 1997). Brain chimeras are obtained by exchanging *in ovo* specific brain areas between embryos of two birds and resulting in hatching chimeric birds. This method applied to the photosensitive fowl led to differentiate the ILS-induced PRs generated by the prosencephalon from those generated by the mesencephalon (Teillet et al., 1991; Guy et al., 1994; Batini et al., 1996):

- <u>Prosencephalic chimeras</u> (having an epileptic prosencephalon grafted on a normal brain). The EEG, at rest, presents continuous PSW and PDs. ILS blocks PSW and PDs and induces EEG desynchronisation, but neither myoclonias nor seizures.

- Mesencephalic chimeras (having an epileptic mesencephalon grafted on a normal brain). The EEG at rest is normal. ILS does not modify the EEG background, does not provoke seizure, but induces neck myoclonias at the ILS frequency which never spread to other structures.
- Promesencephalic chimeras. To obtain generalised myoclonias and generalised seizures, the Fepi grafts need to include both the prosencephalon and the mesencephalon.

Discussion

The comparison of the data concerning the various types of clinical and EEG responses induced by ILS in the three species described above, help to understand the mechanisms of ILS-induced PR generation. It raises, however, some questions for which we do not yet have the answers.

In relation with phylogenesis, some significant results were obtained under ILS. They lead to differentiate between species, and to propose for each of them the cerebral circuits generating the ILS-induced PR.

While in man ILS induces PDs in the FR cortex or PDs and focal seizures in the visual cortex, in Papio papio, PDs and seizures appear only in the FR cortex. This is in favour of the progressive enhancement, in course of the evolution, of the excitability of new cortical areas and circuits which are affected by clinical and EEG PR. The importance, in man, of occipital cortex in the initiation of ILS PDs was demonstrated by experimental (Wilkins et al., 1975) and clinical data (Naquet et al., 1960). However, if the cerebral GABA level is decreased, the Papio papio occipital cortex reacts to ILS in the same manner as in man (visualised as already mentioned) by EEG and clinical seizures (Meldrum et al., 1970).

In fowl, with only an "epileptic" brainstem (as it is experimentally obtained in the mesencephalic chimeras), ILS induces a PR (myoclonia) without EEG PDs. These results demonstrate the importance of the brainstem in this species in the absence of a well-developed neocortex. In fact it should be reminded that the prosencephalon of the birds is not the homologue of the neocortex of the mammals, although in part it has similar sensorimotor functions (Dubbeldam, 1991).

Extrapolating from fowl to man, one is tempted to use these data to confirm the hypothesis of brainstem origin proposed in the early fifties (Gastaut, 1951; Naquet & Batini, 2001) to explain the photomyoclonic response found in old patients (see syndrome 1 in man).

The ILS-induced PR of Papio papio raises other questions:

- Why ILS-induced PDs appearing in the upper part of FR area 6 are associated with eyelid myoclonias, whereas electrical stimulations of this same area evoke movements only in the lower limbs?

- The mode of propagation of ILS-induced myoclonias proceeds from eyelids to face, neck, trunk and therefore follows the same propagation, but in the opposite direction, as that induced in the spinal and brainstem nuclei by somesthetic stimulation (Hallett et al., 1977). This observation is in favour of a brainstem implication in the myoclonias.

For all these reasons, we believe that attributing the ILS-induced myoclonias of Papio papio only to the FR cortex or only to the brainstem is not a sufficient explanation. More likely, both are necessary: the level of excitability and permeability of brainstem circuits seems to be under control of cortical circuits, particularly of the FR areas. This control increases with the phylogenetic corticalisation. Thus the eyelid myoclonias in old men are similar, but not superimposable to the Papio papio eyelid myoclonias. In fact, ILS induces in old men "brainstem" eyelid myoclonias, sometimes followed by FRPDs, "generalised" myoclonias and finally *grand mal* seizures. Moreover, in fowl, the prosencephalon does not control the myoclonias, but facilitates the transition from neck myoclonias to generalised seizures.

Still other problems are not solved.

Why, in man with neurodegenerative disease or in very photosensitive Papio papio, do stimulations outside the "magic" frequencies (*i.e.* isolated or double flashes) generate FRPDs?

- The relations of this type of PR with myoclonias are not very well known. Are they common or exceptional? Are they "generalised" or "focal"? Discrete clinical muscular explorations are necessary for a better knowledge of the relation between clinical and EEG symptoms.

- The mechanisms generating such responses to "isolated" or double flashes are not known. Do they imply a higher permeability of the circuits to the PRs than the "plain" type? In photosensitive Papio papio, GABA antagonists and other convulsant drugs facilitate the appearance of such phenomena. Can their appearance in neurodegenerative diseases have a similar origin? Data on the genetic defects are not conclusive at the present time (Lehesjoki & Koskiniemi, 1999).

- Are the visual afferences sufficient to induce the giant PDs found in the neurodegenerative diseases in man (*see* syndrome 5) and Papio papio (*see* syndrome 1) or do they need summation with nonvisual afferences (*e.g.* somesthetic) induced by the myoclonias itself? In Flaxedil-treated Papio papio, to obtain FRPDs under ILS, injection of substances decreasing the GABA level is needed. In man, no sufficient data are available.

The fact that ILS-induced FRPR do not have the same EEG paroxysmal symptomatology in man, baboon, and chicken raises other problems:

a) Photosensitive epilepsy is usually considered as "generalised epilepsy". The variability of ILS-induced occipital seizures in man, the ILS-induced frontorolandic PDs and seizures in Papio papio, and the ILS-induced brainstem myoclonias and seizures in fowl are opposed to such schematisation.

b) The actual criteria to define what is an "epileptic seizure" are based on electrographic (EEG, extracellular and intracellular unit recording) paroxysmal data. In man, as in Papio papio, ILS-induced myoclonias and seizures are always accompanied by PDs in the EEG but in fowl they are not. The question is therefore: should only the syndromes accompanied by PDs in the EEG or in deep structures be considered as "epileptic"? If myoclonias and seizures not associated with EEG PDs should be considered as "nonepileptic", what is the significance of the paroxysmal EEG at rest as always observed in the "epileptic" fowl?

c) The same questions may be raised, using other types of sensory stimuli.

- Audiogenic seizures: Individual Fepi are affected by both photogenic and audiogenic seizures. In both cases the EEG is paroxysmal at rest and desynchronisation takes place during seizures (Fadlallah et al., 1995). Moreover, rodents with audiogenic seizures have a normal EEG at rest and an arousal reaction during seizures (Faingold et al., 1986; Jobe et al., 1994). Nevertheless, physiologists and particularly pharmacologists consider them as "epileptic". And in fact audiogenic rats and mice are used as an excellent model to test antiepileptic drugs to be administered to human patients (Meldrum, 1984).

- Sensorimotor myoclonias and seizures: Some Papio papio individuals, photosensitive or not, present myoclonias induced by movement. These myoclonias have no EEG expression, neither in cortical surface nor in the deep structures. Moreover, as in other recognised epileptic syndromes, these myoclonias are facilitated by cerebellar lesions (Brailowsky et al., 1975; 1978) and by benzodiazepine administration (Valin et al., 1981) whereas they are well suppressed by anticholinesterase drugs (Rektor et al., 1984; Menini & Naquet, 1986; Menini et al., 1994). In man, some subjects (particularly children and adolescents) present myoclonias (often in bursts) as in the startle disease (Andermann & Andermann, 1986), or seizures as in kinesigenic paroxysmal choreoathetosis (Kertesz, 1967). In both cases, when the origin is genetic, myoclonias and seizures have no EEG expression. They also react, more or less well, to high doses of anticonvulsant drugs. On the other hand, children with other syndromes are considered epileptic only because they have, during sleep, long bursts of PDs without, in some cases, clinical seizures during day or night (Metz-Lutz et al., 2001).

The discussion about the possibility for cerebellar and brainstem circuits to produce "epilepsy" is not recent. Mollica and Naquet (1953) could never obtain a true afterdischarge by electrical stimulation of the cat cerebellum. With the exception of kindling epilepsy, to the best of our knowledge, stimulation of the mammalian brainstem does not produce any true afterdischarge. In our series of investigations in Fayoumi epileptic chicken (Guy et al., 1993), ILS and auditory stimulation never produced electrical seizures (afterdischarge) in the brainstem or in the prosencephalon. On the contrary, they produced EEG desynchronisation, just like the electric stimulation of the brainstem reticular formation in mammalians (Moruzzi & Magoun, 1949). In the beginning of the third millennium, the discussions continue, particularly between neurologists and neuroscientists. There is still no unanimity about what can be called "epileptic" fits. From the data and the discussion presented here, it appears that the problem is particularly interesting in the case of reflex epilepsies, where more than any other form of "epileptic" seizures the brainstem seems to be involved.

At the end of this discussion we would like to pose the question why the ILS *"magic frequency"* is so different between man and baboon, and so close between man and chicken. At this moment, no hypothesis exists to explain these findings. They do not fit into phylogenetic concepts or to the peculiarities of the visual system of man, which are closer to those of the baboon and far from those of the fowl.

■ Acknowledgement

The authors are very grateful to Ray Kado for his help.

References

1. Andermann F, Andermann E. Excessive startle syndromes: startle disease, jumping and startle epilepsy. In: Fahn CD, Marsden MW, eds. *Adv in Neurol*, New York: Raven Press, 1986; 43: 321-38.
2. Artieda J, Obeso JA. The pathology and pharmacology of photic cortical reflex myoclonus. *Ann Neurol* 1993; 34: 175-84.
3. Badinand-Hubert N, Bureau M, Hirsch E, *et al.* Epilepsies and video games: results of a multicentric study. *EEG Clin Neurophysiol* 1998; 107: 422-7.
4. Balzamo E, Bert J, Menini C, Naquet R. Excessive light sensitivity in Papio papio, its variations with age, sex and geographic origin. *Epilepsia* 1975; 16: 269-76.
5. Batini C, Teillet MA, Naquet R, Le Douarin NM. Brain chimeras in birds: application to the study of a genetic form of reflex epilepsy. *Trends Neurosci* 1996; 19: 246-52.
6. Beaumanoir A, Gastaut H, Naquet R, eds. Reflex seizures and reflex epilepsies. *Médecine et Hygiène*. Geneva, 1989; 554.
7. Bickford RG, Sem-Jacobsen CW, White PT, Daly D. Some observations on the mechanism of photic and photometrazol activation. *Electroencephalogr Clin Neurophysiol* 1952; 4: 275-82.
8. Brailowsky S, Menini C, Naquet R. Myoclonus developing after vermisectomy in photosensitive Papio papio. *Electroencephalogr Clin Neurophysiol* 1978; 45: 82-9.
9. Brailowsky S, Silva-Barrat C, Menini Ch, *et al.* Effects of localized, chronic GABA infusion into different cortical areas of the photosensitive baboon Papio papio. *Electroencephalogr Clin Neurophysiol* 1989; 72: 147-56.
10. Brailowsky S, Walter S, Larochelle L, Naquet R. Cervelet et épilepsie photosensible chez le Papio papio: effets de lésions cérébelleuses sur la photosensibilité et les potentiels évoqués visuels. *Rev Electroencephalogr Clin Neurophysiol* 1975; 5: 247-51.
11. Chapman AG. Therapeutic prospects for novel excitatory amino acid antagonists in idiopathic generalized epilepsy. In: Malafosse A, Genton P, Hirsch E, *et al.* eds. *Idiopathic Generalized Epilepsies*. John Libbey, 1994; 463-73.
12. Chapman AG, Meldrum BS. Excitatory amino acid antagonists and epilepsy. *Biochem Soc Trans* 1993; 21: 106-10.
13. Cobb S. Photic driving as a cause of clinical seizures in epileptic patients. *Arch Neurol Psychiat* (Chic.) 1947; 58: 70-1.
14. Crawford RD. Epileptic seizures in domestic fowl. *J Hered* 1970; 61: 185-8.

15. Doose H, Gerken H. On the genetics of EEG-anomalies in childhood. IV Photoconvulsive reaction. *Neuropädiatrie* 1973; 4: 162-71.
16. Doose H, Gerken H, Hien-Volpel, KF, Voelzke E. Genetics of photosensitive epilepsy. *Neuropädiatrie* 1969; 1: 56-73.
17. Dubbeldam JL. The avian and mammalian forebrain: correspondences and differences. In: Andrew RJ, ed. *Neural and behavioural plasticity. The use of the domestic fowl as a model*. Oxford: Oxford Science Publications, 1991; 65-92.
18. Fadlallah N, Guy NTM, Teillet MA, et al. Brain chimeras for the study of an avian model of genetic epilepsy: structures involved in sound and light-induced seizures. *Brain Res* 1995; 675: 55-66.
19. Faingold CL, Travis MA, Gehlbach G, Hoffman WE, et al. Neuronal response abnormalities in the inferior colliculus of the genetically epilepsy-prone rats. *Electroencephalogr Clin Neurophysiol* 1986; 63: 296-305.
20. Fischer-Williams M, Poncet M, Riche D, Naquet R. Light-induced epilepsy in the baboon Papio papio: cortical and depth recordings. *Electroencephalogr Clin Neurophysiol* 1968; 25: 557-69.
21. Fukuda H, Valin A, Bryere P, et al. Role of the forebrain commissure and hemispheric independence in photosensitive response of epileptic baboon Papio papio. *Electroencephalogr Clin Neurophysiol* 1988; 69: 363-70.
22. Fukuda H, Valin A, Menini C, et al. Effect of macular and peripheral Retina coagulation on photosensitive epilepsy in the forebrain bisected baboon Papio papio. *Epilepsia* 1989; 30: 623-30.
23. Gastaut H. Les deux types de réponses photiques irradiées chez l'homme. La décharge myoclonique hypersynchrone et la décharge myoclonique par recrutement. *Rev neurol* 1951; 21: 27-37.
24. Gastaut H, Broughton R. Epileptic seizures. *Clinical and Electrographic Features, Diagnosis and Treatment*. Springfield, Ill: Thomas, 1972; 286.
25. Gastaut H, Trevisan C, Naquet R. Diagnostic value of electroencephalographic abnormalities provoked by intermittent photic stimulation. *Electroencephalogr Clin Neurophysiol* 1958; 10: 94-195.
26. Guy NTM, Batini C, Naquet R, Teillet MA. Avian photogenic epilepsy and embryonic brain chimeras: neuronal activity of the adult prosencephalon and mesencephalon. *Exp Brain Res* 1993; 93: 196-204.
27. Guy N, Teillet MA, Le Gal La Salle G, et al. Genetic epilepsy in chicken, new approaches and concepts. In: Malafosse A, Genton P, Hirsch E, et al. eds. *Idiopathic Generalized Epilepsy*. John Libbey, 1994; 331-948.
28. Guy NTM, Teillet MA, Schuler B, et al. Pattern of electroencephalographic activity during light-induced seizures in genetic epileptic chicken and brain chimeras. *Neurosci Lett* 1992; 145: 55-8.
29. Hallett M, Chadwick D, Adam J, Marsden CD. Reticular reflex myoclonus: a physiological type of human post-hypoxic myoclonus. *J Neurol Neurosurg Psychiatry* 1977; 40: 253-64.
30. Harding GFA, Jeavons PM. Photosensitive Epilepsy. *Clinics in Developmental Medicine* 1994; 33: 182.
31. Jeavons PM. The use of photic stimulation in clinical electroencephalography. *Proc Electroenceph Technol Ass* 1969; 16: 225-40.
32. Jobe PC, Mishra PK, Adams-Curtis Le, et al. The GEPR model of the epilepsies. In: Malafosse A, Genton P, Hirsch E, eds. *Idiopathic Generalized Epilepsy*. John Libbey, 1994; 385-98.
33. Johnson DD, Crichlow EC, Crawford RD. Epileptiform seizures in domestic fowl. IV. The effects of anticonvulsant drugs. *Can J Physiol Pharmacol* 1974; 52: 991-4.
34. Johnson DD, Davis HL. Drug responses and brain biochemistry of the Epi mutant chicken. In: Ookawa T, ed. *The brain and behavior of the fowl*. Japan Scientific Society Press, 1983; 281-96.
35. Kasteleijn-Nolst Trenité DGA. Photosensitivity in epilepsy. Electrophysiological and clinical correlates. *Acta Neurol Scand* 1989; 80 (suppl. 125): 3-149.

36. Kasteleijn-Nolst Trenité DGA, Van Emde Boas W, Binnie CD. Photosensitivity. A human model of epilepsy. In: Malafosse A, Genton P, Hirsch E, et al. eds. *Idiopathic Generalized Epilepsies*. John Libbey, 1994; 297-303.

37. Kertesz A. Paroxysmal kinesigenic choreoathetosis. *Neurology* 1967; 17: 680-90.

38. Killam KF, Killam EK, Naquet R. Mise en évidence chez certains singes d'un syndrome myoclonique. *C R Acad Sci* (Paris) 1966a; 262: 1010-2.

39. Killam KF, Naquet R, Bert J. Paroxysmal responses to intermittent light in a population of baboons (Papio papios). *Epilepsia* (Amst) 1966b; 7: 215-9.

40. Killam KF, Killam EK, Naquet R. An animal model of light sensitive epilepsy. *Electroencephalogr Clin Neurophysiol* 1967; 22: 497-513.

41. Klass DW, Fischer-Williams M. Sensory stimulation, sleep and sleep deprivation. In: Remond A, ed. *Handbook of EEG Vol. 1B*. Amsterdam: Elsevier, 1976; 5-73.

42. Kooi KA, Thomas MH, Mortenson F. Photoconvulsive and Photomyoclonic responses in adults. *Neurol* (Minneapolis) 1960; 10: 1051-8.

43. Le Douarin NM. Particularités du noyau interphasique chez la caille japonnaise (Coturnix coturnix japonica). Utilisation de ces particularités comme "marquage biologique" dans les recherches sur les interactions tissulaires et les migrations cellulaires au cours de l'ontogenèse. *Bull Biol Fr Belg* 1969; 103: 435-52.

44. Le Douarin NM. Embryonic neural chimeras in the study of brain development. *Trens Neurosci* 1993; 16: 64-72.

45. Le Douarin NM, Catala M, Batini C. Embryonic neural chimeras in the study of vertebrate brain and head development. *Intern Rev Cythology* 1997; 175: 241-309.

46. Lehesjoki AE, Koskiniemi M. Progressive Myoclonus Epilepsy of Unverricht-Lundborg Type. *Epilepsia* 1999; 40 (suppl. 3): 23-8.

47. Lloyd-Smith DL, Henderson LR. Epileptic patients showing susceptibility to photic stimulation alone. *Electroencephalogr Clin Neurophysiol* 1951; 3: 378-9.

48. Meldrum BS. Amino acid neurotransmitters and new approaches to anticonvulsant drug action. *Epilepsia* 1984; 25 (suppl. 2): S140-9.

49. Meldrum BS, Balzamo E, Gadea M, Naquet R. Photic and drug-induced epilepsy in the baboon (Papio papio). The effect of isoniazid, thiosemi-carbazide, pyridoxine and amino-oxyacetic acid. *Electroencephalogr Clin Neuro-physiol* 1970; 29: 333-47.

50. Ménini C, Naquet R. Les Myoclonies. Des myoclonies du Papio papio à certaines myoclonies humaines. *Rev Neurol* 1986; 142: 3-28.

51. Menini C, Silva-Barrat C, Naquet R. The epileptic and nonepileptic generalized myoclonus of the Papio papio baboon. In: Malafosse A, Genton P, Hirsch E, eds. *Idiopathic Generalized Epilepsies*. John Libbey, 1994; 331-48.

52. Menini C, Stutzmann JM, Laurent H, Naquet R. Paroxysmal visual evoked potentials (PVEPs) in the *Papio papio*. I Morphological and topographical characteristics. Comparison with paroxysmal discharges. *Electroencephalogr Clin Neurophysiol* 1980; 50: 356-64.

53. Metz-Lutz MA, Maquet P, Saint-Martin A de, et al. Pathophysiological aspects of Landau-Kleffner syndrome: From the active epileptic phase to recovery. In: Engel J Jr, Schwartzkroin PA, Moshe SL, Lowenstein DH, eds. *Brain Plasticity and Epilepsy*. Academic Press, 2001; 505-26.

54. Mollica A, Naquet R. Activité convulsive et silence électrique dans l'écorce cérébelleuse. *Electroencephalogr Clin Neurophysiol* 1953; 5: 585-7.

55. Moruzzi G, Magoun HW. Brainstem reticular formation and activation of the EEG. *Electroencephalogr Clin Neurophysiol* 1949; 1: 455-73.

56. Naquet R. Contribution of experimental epilepsy to understanding some particular forms in man. In: Brazier MAB, ed. *Epilepsy, its phenomenon in man*. New York: Academic Press, 1973; 37-65.

57. Naquet R. Genetic study of epilepsy in contributions of different models especially the photosensitive Papio papio. In: Brazier MAB, ed. *Growth and development of the Brain*. New York: Rave Press, 1975; 219-30.
58. Naquet R, Batini C. Genetic reflex epilepsy. In: *Epilepsy and Movement Disorders*. Guerrini R, Aicardi J, Andermann F, Hallett M (eds). Cambridge University Press, 2002: 557.
59. Naquet R, Fegersten L, Bert J. Seizure discharges localized to the posterior cerebral regions in man, provoked by intermittent photic stimulation. *Electroencephalogr Clin Neurophysiol* 1960; 16: 140-52.
60. Naquet R, Meldrum BS. Myoclonus induced by intermittent light stimulation in the baboon. Neurophysiological and Neuropharmacological approaches. *Advances in Neurology* 1985; 43: 611-27.
61. Naquet R, Menini C, Catier J. Photically induced epilepsy in Papio papio. The initiation of discharges and the role of the frontal cortex and of the corpus callosum. In: Brazier MAB, Petsche H, eds. *Synchronisation of the EEG in the epilepsy*. Vienna: Springer, 1972; 347-67.
62. Naquet R, Poncet-Ramade M. Paroxysmal discharges induced by intermittent light stimulation. In: *Henri Gastaut and the Marseilles School's to the Neurosciences (EEG Suppl. No. 35)*, Broughton RJ, ed. Amsterdam: Elsevier Biomedical Press, 1982; 447.
63. Naquet R, Valin A. Experimental Models of Reflex Epilepsy. Reflex Epilepsies and Reflex Seizures. In: Zifkin BG, Andermann F, Beaumanoir A, Rowan JR, eds. *Advances in Neurology Vol. 75*. Philadelphia: Lippincott-Raven Publishers, 1998; 15-28.
64. Naquet R, Wada JA. Role of the corpus callosum in photosensitive seizures of epileptic baboon Papio papio. *Adv Neurol* 1992; 57: 579-87.
65. Nekhorocheff MI. La stimulation lumineuse intermittente chez l'enfant normal. *Rev Neurol* (Paris) 1950; 83: 601-2.
66. Newmark ME, Penry JK. Photosensitivity and Epilepsy: a Review. New York: Raven Press, 1979; 220.
67. Panayotopoulos CP, Jeavons PM, Harding GFA. Occipital spikes and their relation to visual evoked responses in epilepsy, with particular reference to photosensitive epilepsy. *EEG Clin Neurophysiol* 1972; 32: 179-90.
68. Rektor I, Bryere P, Valin A, *et al*. Physostigmine antagonizes the benzodiazepine-induced myoclonus in the baboon Papio papio. *Neuirosci-Lett* 1984; 52: 91-6.
69. Robertson EG. Photogenic epilepsy self-precipitated attacks. *Brain* 1954; 77: 232-51.
70. Teillet MA, Naquet R, Le Gal La Salle G, *et al*. Transfer of genetic epilepsy by embryonic brain grafts in the chicken. *Proc Natl Acad Sci USA* 1991; 88: 6966-70.
71. Valin A, Cepeda C, Rey E, Naquet R. Opposite effects of clorazepam on two kinds of myoclonus in the photosensitive Papio papio. *Electroencephalogr Clin Neurophysiol* 1981; 52: 647-51.
72. Walter WG, Walter VJ, Gastaut H, Gastaut Y. Une forme électroencéphalographique nouvelle de l'épilepsie: L'épilepsie photogénique. *Rev Neurol* 1948; 80: 613-4.
73. Waltz S. Photosensitivity and epilepsy: a genetic approach. In: Malafosse A, Genton P, Hirsch E, *et al*. eds. *Idiopathic Generalized Epilepsy*. John Libbey, 1994; 317-28.
74. Wilkins AJ, Andermann F, Ives J. Stripes, complex cells and seizures. *Brain* 1975; 98: 365-80.

Prevention of photosensitive seizures by optical filters

Y. Takahashi[1], S. Fujiwara[2], N. Matsuo, S. Hattori, M. Ariki, T. Sato[3]

*Department of Pediatrics, Gifu Prefectural Gifu Hospital,
4-6-1 Noishiki Gifu 500-8717, Japan
[1]National Epilepsy Center, Shizuoka Institute of Epilepsy and Neurological Disorders, 886 Urushiyama, Shizuoka, 420-8688, Japan
[2]Filtec Inc., 1214-1-614 Kunugida-cho Hatiouji, Tokyo 193-0942, Japan
[3]Faculty of Textile Science, Kyoto Institute of Technology, Goshokaido-cho, Matsugasaki, Sakyo-ku, Kyoto 606-8585, Japan*

Introduction

As television has become virtually a universal source of information and entertainment, televised images are the most common stimulus for provoking photosensitive seizures. In Europe, more than 60% of photosensitive epileptic patients experienced their first photosensitive seizure while watching television (Harding & Jeavons, 1994). In Japan, in December 1997, the animated TV program "Pocket Monsters" simultaneously induced seizures in photosensitive persons all over the country, and several hundred viewers were rushed to emergency hospitals *(Table I)*. This event served as a warning that the artificial light from televised images could accidentally induce seizures in photosensitive persons. In addition, because 76% of the affected viewers had latent photosensitivity, that is, they were unaware of their risk for light-induced seizures, and had never before experienced epileptic seizures (Takahashi *et al.*, 1999a), the incident also brought attention to the prevalence of photosensitivity in nonepileptic persons in Japan. The prevalence of nonepileptic photosensitivity ranges from 0.5%-8.9% of the world's population (Buchthal & Lennox, 1953; Doose & Waltz, 1993; Eeg-Olofsson *et al.*, 1971; Gregory *et al.*, 1993; Kooi *et al.*, 1960; Mundy-Castle, 1953), and is higher around the age of puberty (Harding & Fylan, 1999). The evolution of photosensitivity is an age-dependent phenomenon *(Figure 1)*.

Emission from red fluorescents of the normal cathode ray tube (CRT) has a peak at ~ 706 nm, which causes mono-cone (L-cone) stimulation and leads to induction of the photoparoxysmal response (PPR) (Takahashi *et al.*, 1995b) *(Figure 2)*. This characteristic emission at ~ 706 nm seems to contribute to the induction of

Table I. Summary of "Pocket Monsters" incident

- Audience rate: 16.5%* (43.7% of viewers from 6-18 years old)
- All symptoms: 10.4% of viewers
- Seizures
  - 1.8% of viewers (Metropolitan district)
  - 0.02% of viewers (Aichi prefecture)
  - 0.0044% of viewers (Kantou district)
  - ≤ 76% of viewers had never before experienced epileptic seizures or photosensitive seizures (Gifu district)
- Eye pain: 4.2% of viewers (school based)
- Nausea: 1.5% of viewers (school based)
- Headache: 0.3% of viewers (school based)

* Number in population viewing the program divided by the number in the population.
Compiled from Ebata et al., 1998; Furusho et al., 1998; Takada et al., 1999; Takahashi et al., 1999a.

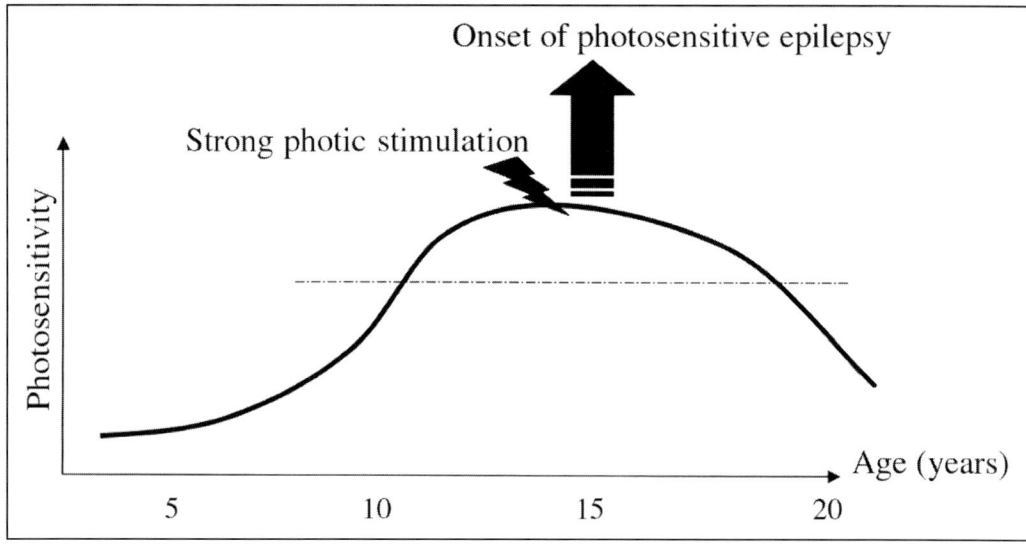

Figure 1. Evolution of photosensitivity. Photosensitivity runs an age-dependent course, with the incidence increasing from approximately 10 years of age, reaching a peak at puberty, and decreasing to approximately 20 years of age. Photosensitivity is a predispositional condition and cannot be recognized before the occurrence of photosensitive seizures or by chance EEG examination. The prevalence of nonepileptic photosensitivity seems to be 20-fold that of epileptic photosensitivity. Many nonepileptic persons with latent photosensitivity never have photosensitive seizures, but some become highly photosensitive and often have seizures after chance exposure to strong photic stimulation, such as from TV viewing, resulting in the onset of photosensitive epilepsy.

photosensitive seizures by TV viewing. Furthermore, some TVs have an abnormally high emission of long-wavelength red light (Takahashi et al., 2001), which is essential for the PPR. In the "Pocket Monsters" incident, the majority of TVs that induced seizures emitted a higher level of long-wavelength red light than TVs that did not induce seizures in photosensitive viewers (*Figure 3*). We have estimated that a higher emission of long-wavelength red light stimulated the wavelength-dependent

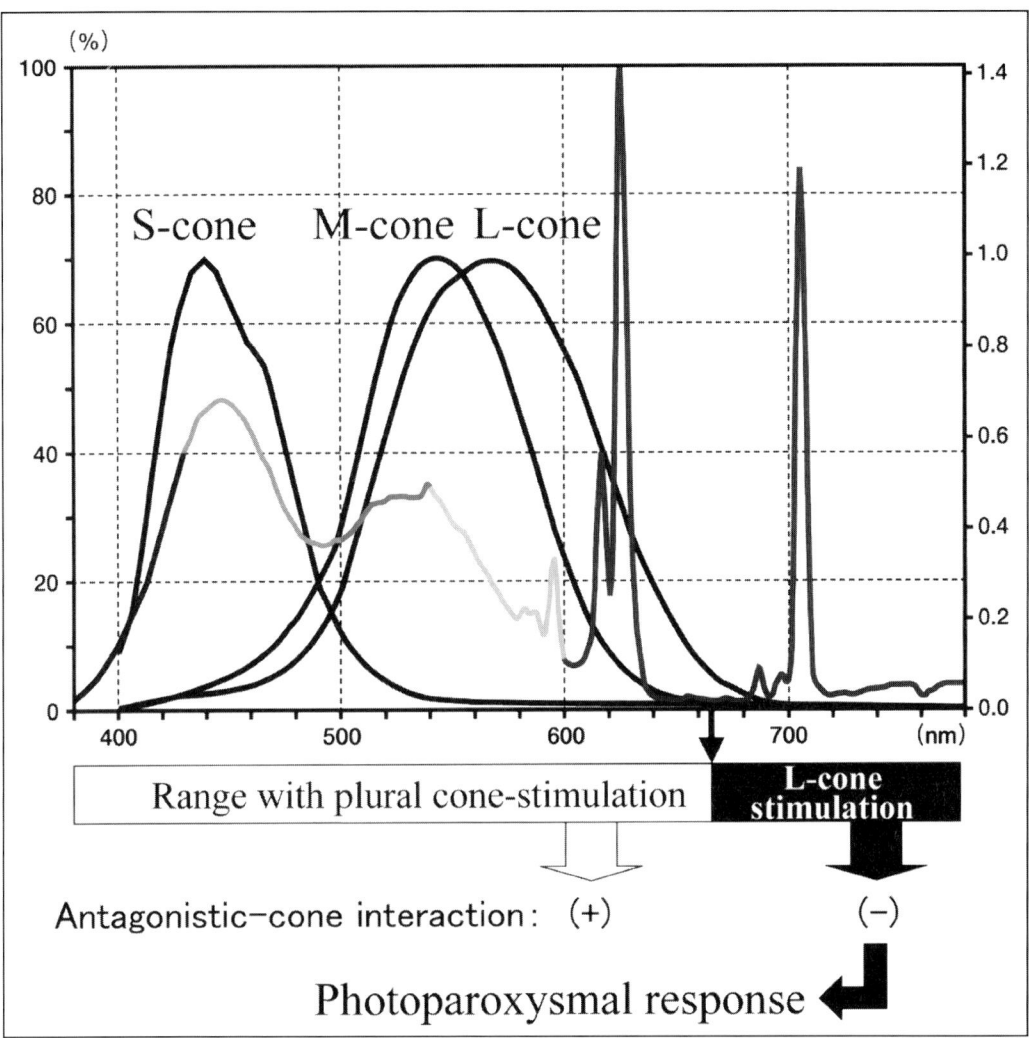

Figure 2. Mono-cone stimulation by long-wavelength red light. Black lines indicate relative sensitivities of three retinal cones (scale on the right vertical axis). Colored line indicates normal emission of three fluorescents on white color bar of CRTs (scale on left vertical axis). Peak luminance energy in the visible range is shown as 100%. The horizontal axis shows the wavelength (nm). Red fluorescents have two emission peaks on ~ 627 nm and ~ 706 nm, and green fluorescents have an emission peak on ~ 545 nm, and blue fluorescents have an emission peak on ~ 450 nm. Light in the visible range longer than ~ 670 nm stimulates L-cones only, resulting in mono-cone stimulation without antagonistic-cone interaction in retinal ganglion cells.

mechanism of photosensitivity (Takahashi et al., 1995b; 1997a, b; 1999b, c) and played an important role in the induction of photosensitive seizures (Figure 2). We are concerned about the existence of TVs in the community with an abnormally high emission of long-wavelength red light and the increase of intrinsic photosensitivity in photosensitive persons from daily watching of such TVs. Thus, we believe that it

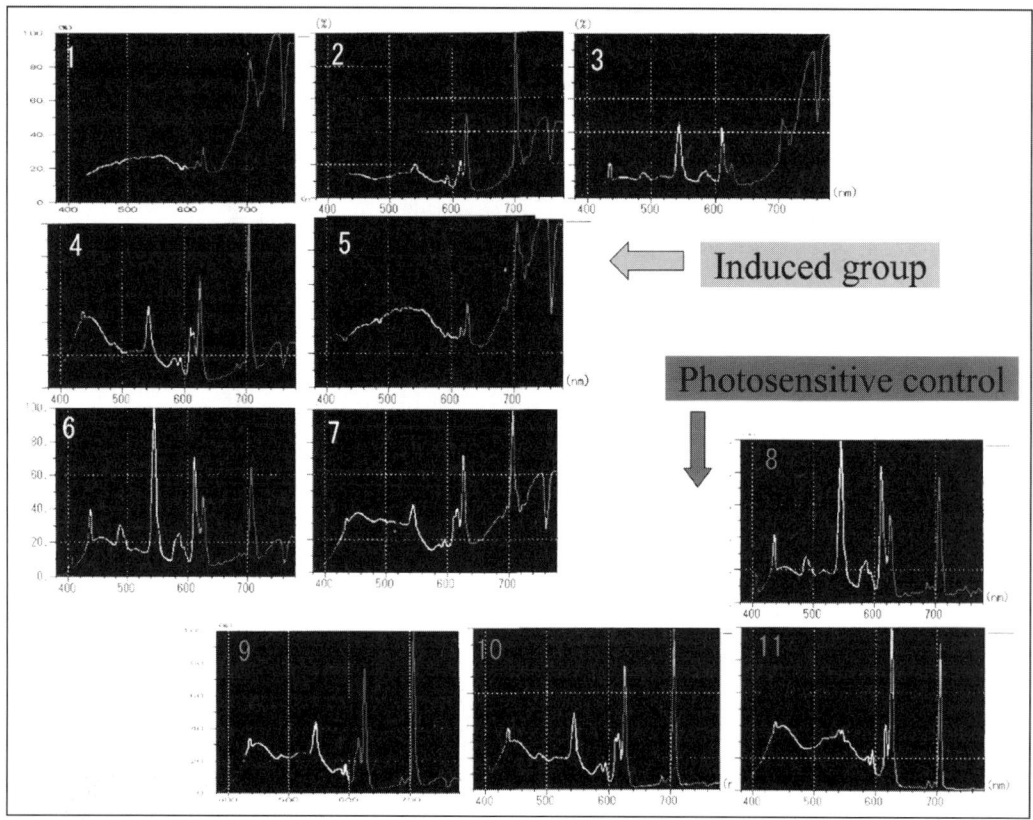

Figure 3. Emission patterns of the CRTs. Numbers indicate the patient and CRT. Luminance energy [w/(sr m² nm)] from 380 to 780 nm was measured by the spectroradiometer (Minolta CS1000) in the black portion of the color bar on the CRTs, and peak luminance energy in the visible range is shown as 100% in each panel. The horizontal axis shows the wavelength (nm). In the "Pocket Monsters" incident, some photosensitive viewers had seizures (induced group) but others did not have seizures (photosensitive control) while watching the program. A majority of the TVs of the induced group emitted a higher level of long-wavelength red light longer than 710 nm than TVs of photosensitive controls. The abnormal emission of long-wavelength red light might be causally related to the heating of shadow masks in the CRTs.

is necessary to establish a universal prophylactic strategy against TV-induced seizures, not only for photosensitive epileptic patients, but also for persons with latent photosensitivity who are naive about their risk for light-induced seizures.

Using intermittent photic stimulation (IPS) and wavelength-specific optical filters, and following the mono-cone stimulation theory (Binnie et al., 1984), we have identified two different pathophysiological mechanisms of the PPR (Takahashi et al., 1995b; 1997a, b; 1999b, c). One is a wavelength-dependent mechanism, in which PPRs are elicited only when the flashing light contains long-wavelength red light longer than ~ 670 nm (Figure 2). Long-wavelength red light (a normal peak at 706 nm from red fluorescents and abnormal emission from heated shadow masks) stimulates L-cones only, resulting in the absence of an antagonistic-cone interaction at the retinal ganglion cells (Takahashi et al., 1995b). The other mechanism depends only on the quantity of light required for eliciting PPRs, and is independent of the wavelength-composition of the flashing light (Takahashi et al., 1997b; 1999b, c). Taking into consideration the two different pathophysiological mechanisms, the existence of latent photosensitivity, the emission of red fluorescents at ~ 706 nm, and the abnormal emission of long-wavelength red light from shadow masks in some TVs, we designed novel, special optical filters to inhibit PPRs. The goal was to prevent photosensitive seizures by a nonpharmacological, universal method for reducing the level of photic stimulation from televised images before they reach the retina.

Patients and methods

Informed consent was obtained by the method prescribed by the ethical committee of Gifu University School of Medicine or Gifu Prefectural Gifu Hospital. We studied 14 photosensitive epileptic patients who had idiopathic generalised epilepsy, occipital lobe epilepsy, or epilepsy with continuous spike and wave discharges during slow-wave sleep, and two photosensitive nonepileptic patients who had febrile convulsions (Table II). The photosensitive epileptic and nonepileptic patients had classic PPRs to conventional IPS during EEG examination. Classic PPR was defined as the reliable PPR described by Klass and Fischer-Williams (1976) and Binnie et al. (1986). All participants were normal trichromats, according to the Ishihara test. Mean age at examination was 13.1 ± 3.2 years (n = 18) for the epileptic patients and 5.7 ± 1.7 years (n = 3) for the nonepileptic patients. (Five subjects each had two examinations.) Three of the epileptic patients who were examined before treatment with antiepileptic drugs tended to have PPRs to a relatively wide range of flash frequencies.

Conventional IPS, with a Grass PS22 or PS33 photic stimulator, was performed under the following conditions: flash intensity, 8; flash duration, 10 micro s; flash rate, 1-30 Hz; and a flash lamp placed 30 cm from the nasion (Klass & Fischer-Williams, 1976; Takahashi et al., 1995b; 1997a, b; 1999b, c). The examinations to determine the effects of optical filters on the inhibition of PPRs were performed in a darkened-shielded room. The optical filters were purchased from Filtec (Tokyo, Japan). TF1 and TF2 are specially made optical filters that do not transmit long-wavelength red light. ND50 and ND70 are neutral density filters that evenly absorb light in the visible spectrum. CM500 is a color-compensating filter. V10 and V30 are multiband calibration filters. TF270, TF250, and TF2V3 are compound filters composed of TF2 and ND70, ND50, or V30. TF170, TF150, TF1V3, and TF1V1 are compound filters composed of TF1 and ND70, ND50, V30, or V10. CMV1 and CMV3 are compound filters composed of CM500 and V10 or V30. Testing with the optical filters was carried out at the flash frequency that had elicited the most prominent PPRs to conventional IPS with the eyes open. The flash frequency was 18 Hz, except in patients 2, 4, 5, 11, 14, and 15, where it was 15 Hz, and in patients 7 and 10, where it was 21 Hz. The optical filters were fixed in front of, and completely covered, the eyes. The quantity, luminance, and chromaticity of the flashing light, with and without filters, were measured by a spectroradiometer (Minolta CS1000, Minolta, Japan).

Table II. Optical filters and photoparoxysmal response in photosensitive epileptic and nonepileptic patients

Patient	Diagnosis	Age (yr)	AED	IPS (Hz)	TF2	TF270	TF250	TF2V3	TF170	TF150	TF1V3	TF1V1	CMV1	CMV3	ND50	ND70
1	IGE	10	None	12-30	+	+	–	+	–	–	–	NT	NT	NT	NT	NT
2	IGE	13	VPA	15	NT	–	–	–	–	–	–	NT	NT	NT	NT	NT
3	IGE	13	VPA	15	–	–	–	–	–	–	–	–	–	–	–	–
3	IGE	14	VPA	12-21	NT	–	–	–	–	–	–	NT	NT	NT	NT	NT
	IGE	15	VPA	12-18	+	+	–	+	+	–	–	–	–	–	–	–
4	IGE	16	None	12-21	+	–	–	–	+	–	–	–	–	–	+	–
5	IGE	18	VPA	15	+	–	–	+	–	–	–	–	–	–	+	–
6	OLE	5	PHT	21	–	–	–	–	–	–	–	NT	–	–	–	NT
7	OLE	11	VPA	18-21	NT	+	+	+	–	–	–	NT	NT	NT	NT	NT
	OLE	11	VPA	9-30	+	+	+	+	+	–	–	–	+	+	–	–
8	OLE	11	CBZ	18	–	–	–	–	–	–	–	NT	NT	NT	NT	NT
9	OLE	11	CBZ	15-30	–	–	–	–	–	–	–	NT	NT	NT	NT	NT
10	OLE	11	None	6-30	+	+	+	+	–	+	+	+	–	–	+	+
11	OLE	14	VPA	12-30	–	–	+	+	–	–	–	NT	NT	NT	NT	NT
12	OLE	14	VPA	15-21	+	+	–	+	–	+	–	NT	NT	NT	NT	NT
13	OLE	18	VPA	21	NT	–	–	–	–	–	–	NT	NT	NT	NT	NT
	OLE	18	VPA	15-18	+	+	+	–	–	–	+	–	–	–	–	–
14	CSWS	13	PHT	9-21	–	–	+	–	–	–	–	–	–	–	–	+
15	NE	4	None	6-30	+	–	–	–	–	–	–	NT	NT	NT	NT	NT
15	NE	5	None	9-18	–	+	+	+	–	–	–	–	–	+	+	+
16	NE	8	None	15-21	–	–	–	–	–	–	–	NT	–	–	NT	NT
Rate of transmission (%)*					63.6	48.7	28.5	20.7	43.2	24.4	15.5	30.2	28.8	14.8	38.2	53.3
Rate of inhibition (%)†					52.9	61.9	66.7	57.1	85.7	85.7	90.5	90.0	90.9	81.8	33.3	50.0

AED: antiepileptic drug; CBZ: carbamazepine; CSWS: continuous spike and wave discharges in slow-wave sleep; IGE: idiopathic generalised epilepsy; IPS: intermittent photic stimulation; NE: nonepileptic subject; NT: not tested; OLE: occipital lobe epilepsy; PHT: phenytoin; VPA: valproic acid.
Age means age at time of examination.
Plus sign (+) indicates that the PPR was not inhibited by the optical filter.
Minus sign (–) indicates that the PPR was inhibited by the optical filter.
* Ratio of luminance of the white color bar on the cathode ray tube with and without optical filters.
† Inhibition rate of PPRs (number of examinations without PPRs divided by total number of examinations).

Results

The optical filters eliciting or inhibiting PPRs and their transmission and calculated inhibition rates are shown in *Table II*. The effects of the optical filters were inconsistent in some patients. That is, some filters could inhibit PPRs, at the stage when PPRs were elicited by a narrow range of flash frequencies, indicating a low level of photosensitivity, but could not inhibit PPRs, when PPRs were elicited by a wider range of flash frequencies, indicating a high level of photosensitivity.

TF2, which reflects and does not transmit long-wavelength red light *(Figure 4)*, inhibited PPRs in 52.9% of the examinations. The neutral density filters, which almost evenly absorb light in the visible spectrum *(Figure 4)*, inhibited PPRs in one-third to one-half of the examinations.

Compound filters, composed of filters reflecting long-wavelength red light and neutral density filters, inhibited PPRs in 57.1%-90.9% of the examinations *(Table II)*. The inhibition rates of the compound filters were higher than those of either the filters reflecting long-wavelength red light or the neutral density filters. The inhibition rates of the compound filters TF2, TF250, and TF270 were in the order of TF2 < TF270 < TF250 (N.S.) *(Figure 5)*. Comparing the data of filters with different levels of reflection of long-wavelength red light, inhibition rates of compound filters were in the order of ND70 < TF270 < TF170 and ND50 < TF250 < TF150 ($p = 0.02$ and $p = 0.008$, respectively; both Mann-Whitney's U test) *(Figure 6)*. These comparisons showed that the reduction of long-wavelength red light had a significant inhibitory effect on PPRs. Compound filters based on TF1, which reflects more long-wavelength red light, strongly inhibited PPRs *(Figure 7)*. The compound filters composed of TF1 and multiband calibration filters inhibited PPRs in 90% of examinations. Filters TF170, TF1V1, and CMV1 had superior inhibitory properties, with an inhibition rate of more than 85% and a transmission rate of more than 25%.

On spectroradiometry, the white color bar on the CRT emitted four main peaks: long-wavelength red at ~ 706 nm, red at ~ 627 nm, green at ~ 545 nm, and blue at ~ 450 nm *(Figures 3 and 8A)*, and the chromaticity diagram of the white color bar was exactly on white. Spectroradiometry results and the chromaticity diagram of the optical filters with an inhibition rate of more than 85% (compound filters CMV1, TF1V3, TF1V1, TF170, TF150) are shown in *Figures 8B-F*. Filter CMV1, which had the most efficient rate of PPR inhibition, absorbed the long-wavelength red peak completely, and the other peaks partially. Chromaticity of the white color bar viewed through CMV1 deviated slightly toward green from white. CMV1 failed to inhibit PPRs only when there was a high level of photosensitivity (patient 7). TF1V3 had a good inhibition rate, but a low transmission rate. TF1V1, which reflected more red light and had a higher transmission rate than CMV1, had a good inhibition rate, equal to that of CMV1. With TF1V1, PPRs were observed only in the absence of antiepileptic drug treatment and when there was a high level of photosensitivity (patient 10). Although TF170 and TF150 reflected a large part of the red peak, TF170 and TF150 adequately spared the green and blue peaks *(Figure 8)*. TF170 had the

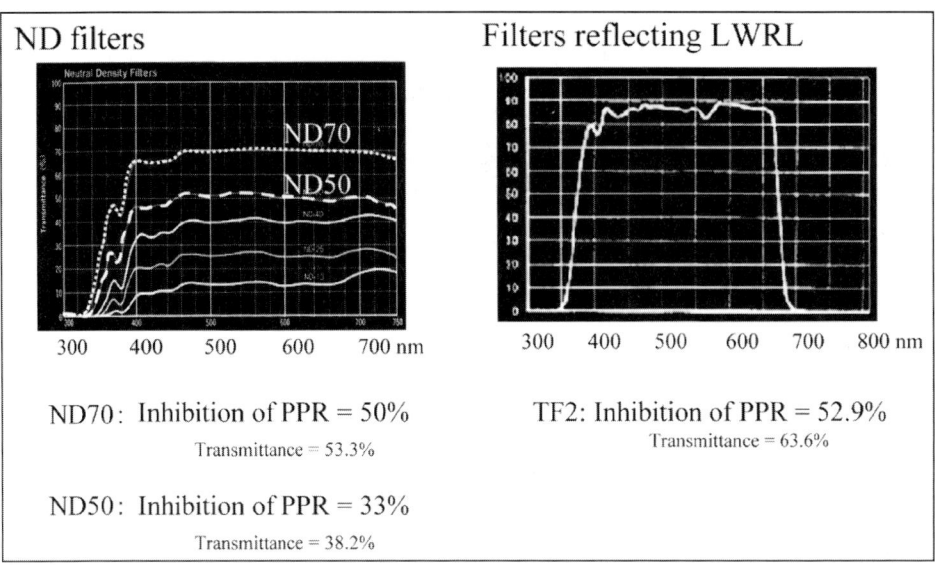

Figure 4. Optical characteristics of neutral density (ND) filters, filters reflecting long-wavelength red light (LWRL) and inhibition of PPRs. The vertical axis shows transmission spectra (%) and the horizontal axis shows the wavelength (nm) in each panel (also for Figs. 5, 6, and 7). ND70 and ND50 evenly absorbed 30% and 50%, respectively, of light in the visible spectrum.

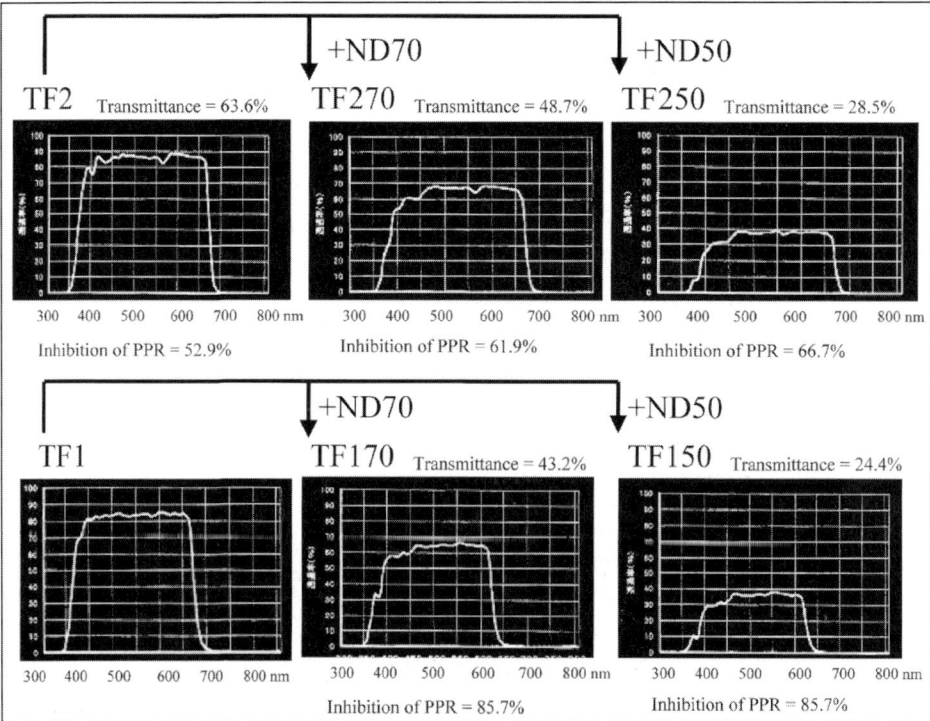

Figure 5. Optical characteristics and inhibition of compound optical filters. Upper panels show data of compound optical filters based on TF2; lower panels show data of filters based on TF1.

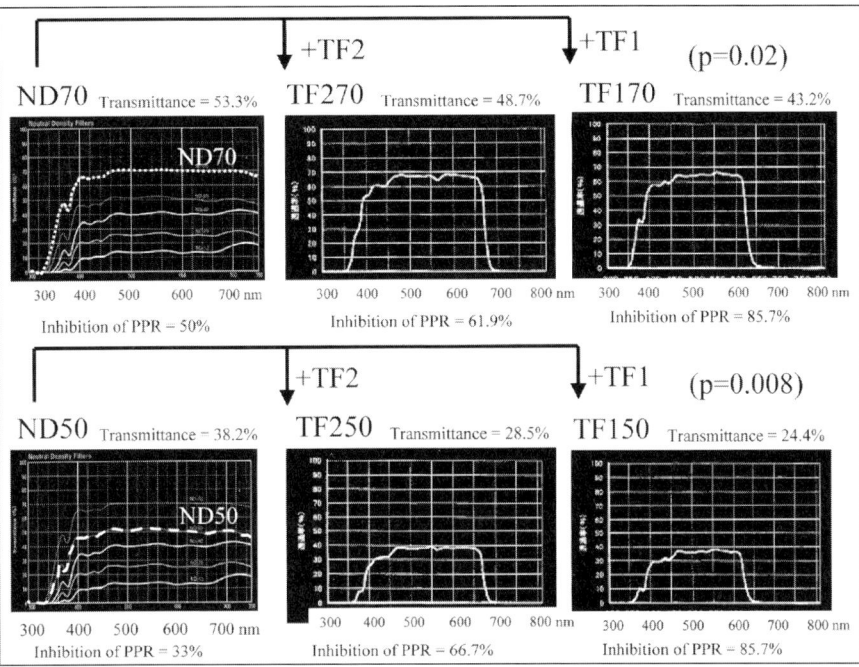

Figure 6. Optical characteristics and inhibition of compound optical filters. Upper panels show data of compound optical filters based on ND70; lower panels show data of filters based on ND50.

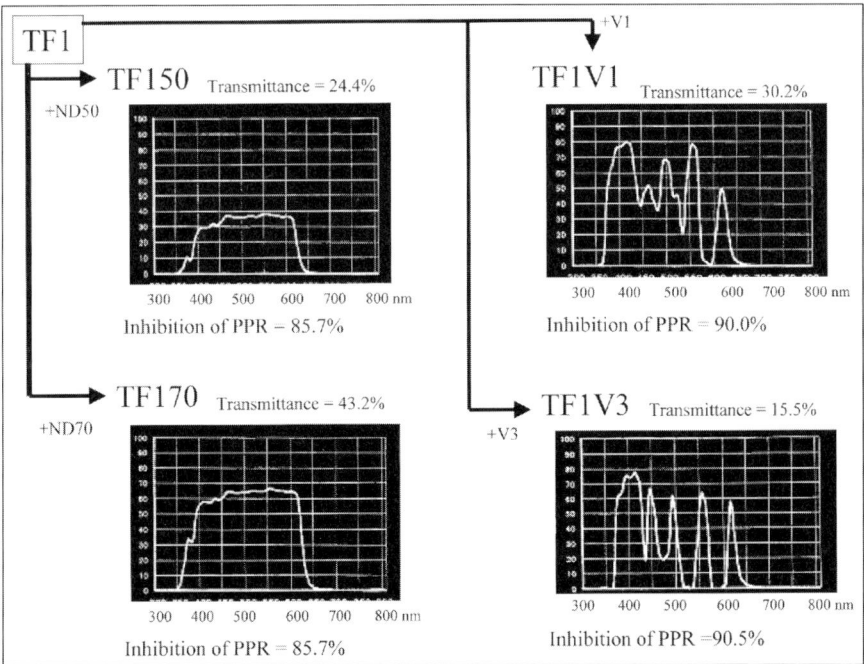

Figure 7. Optical characteristics and inhibition of compound optical filters composed of TF1 and neutral density filters or multiband calibration filters.

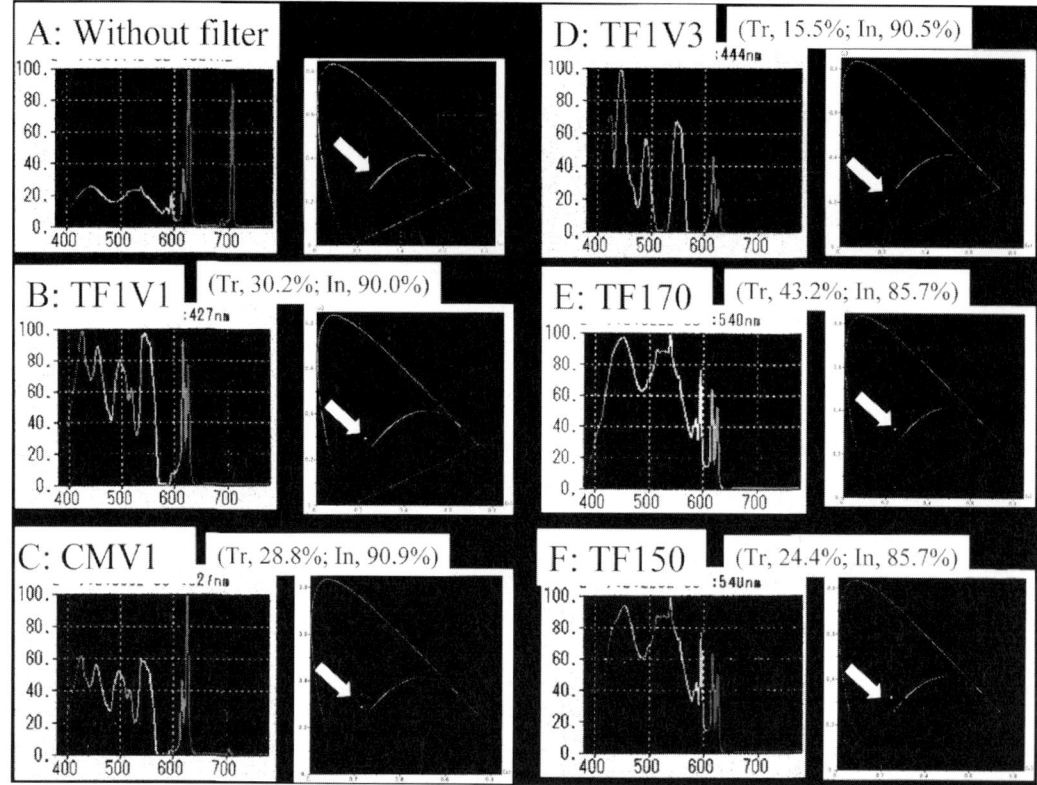

Figure 8. Spectroradiometry and chromaticity diagram of white images on CRT with and without optical filters. In all panels (A-F), spectroradiometry data are shown on the left, and chromaticity diagrams are shown on the right. On the spectroradiometry graphs, the vertical axis shows the ratio of emission from CRT (%), and peak luminance energy in the visible range is shown as 100%; the horizontal axis shows the wavelength (nm). On the chromaticity diagrams, the vertical axis shows y and the horizontal axis x on the xy-color expression system. Tr: ratio of luminance with filters to that without filters; In: inhibition rate of PPRs by the filter.

highest transmission rate among the five filters. There was minimal modification of chromaticity by the compound optical filters. In nonepileptic subjects, CMV1, TF1V1, and TF170 all inhibited the PPRs.

■ Discussion

We have shown that optical filters reflecting long-wavelength red light or neutral density optical filters are inadequate for inhibiting PPRs, and that compound filters (composed of filters reflecting long-wavelength red light and neutral density filters) inhibit approximately 90% of PPRs. These results suggest that the induction of PPRs has two pathophysiological mechanisms operating in a parallel manner. Either a wavelength-dependent mechanism or a quantity-of-light-dependent mechanism of photosensitivity (Takahashi et al., 1995b; 1997a, b; 1999b, c) contributes to the induction of PPRs. The customary optical filters (dark glasses) need absorption of 90% to provide some protection against photosensitivity (Binnie & Jeavons, 1992), but our compound filters, with far less absorption, provide almost complete protection against PPRs in photosensitive persons, regardless of whether they have epilepsy or not. Absorption of long-wavelength red light seems to play an important role in the inhibition of PPRs.

Because PPRs are usually a seizure-preceding event, we suppose that the inhibition of PPRs would result in the prophylaxis of photosensitive seizures. The inhibition rate of some compound filters was approximately 90% with examination at a close distance (30 cm from the strobe light to the nasion). Television viewing is usually done at a distance of approximately 1.5 m. Therefore, we estimate that the PPRs and succeeding photosensitive seizures can be abolished by the use of compound filters while watching TV. The good color balance on the chromaticity diagram, as well as the good transmission and PPR inhibition rates, qualify the compound filters CMV1, TF1V1, and TF170 for daily TV viewing.

The induction of photosensitive seizures is defined by the relative balance between photosensitivity and photic stimulation. That is, in persons with a lower level of photosensitivity, only stronger photic stimulation can induce seizures, and in those with a higher level of photosensitivity, weaker photic stimulation can be enough for induction. The balance can be affected by several factors that modulate photosensitivity and photic stimulation (*Figure 9*). The photosensitivity level is modulated by the subject's age, health condition (*e.g.* infection, somnolence), and antiepileptic drug therapy, and probably by daily exposure to long-wavelength red light from TV viewing. Photic stimulation levels are modulated by the quantity of long-wavelength red light emitted from the TV, viewing distance from the TV, contrast of images on CRT, type of electric-wave receiving system, and ambient lighting during TV viewing (Takahashi et al., 1999a).

Decreasing the level of photosensitivity or photic stimulation could lead to the prevention of photosensitive seizures. Although the customary treatment for photosensitive epileptic seizures is antiepileptic drugs, which reduce photosensitivity, our optical filters offer an alternative, nonpharmacological means of reducing photic stimulation, permitting the effective management of photosensitivity. Moreover, the successive daily use of blue-tinted contact lens to reduce photosensitivity in an infant with severe myoclonic epilepsy (Takahashi et al., 1995a) suggests that the daily use of compound optical filters might ameliorate the age-dependent increase of photosensitivity.

In persons with latent photosensitivity and in photosensitive epileptic patients, our compound optical filters can prevent the occurrence or recurrence of photosensitive seizures, resulting in a better quality of life (job or driver's license), as well as the possibility of entertainment with safe images on TV, and education with safe images on the CRT of a personal computer (*Figure 10*). Because photosensitive nonepileptic persons are unaware of their risk for seizures, antiepileptic medication is not an option for preventing photosensitive seizures. These persons, whose prevalence is approximately 9% in children (Doose & Waltz, 1993), can benefit from the ability of our compound filters to inhibit PPRs to chance strong photic stimulation from TV, even those that emit high levels of long-wavelength red light. This practice might

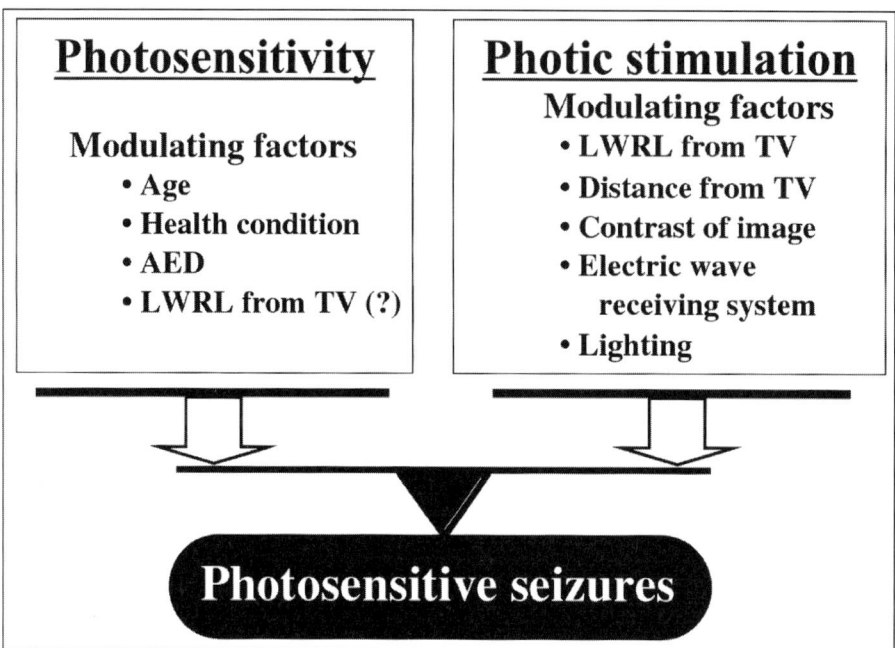

Figure 9. Factors modulating photosensitivity and photic stimulation. AED: antiepileptic drugs; LWRL: long-wavelength red light.

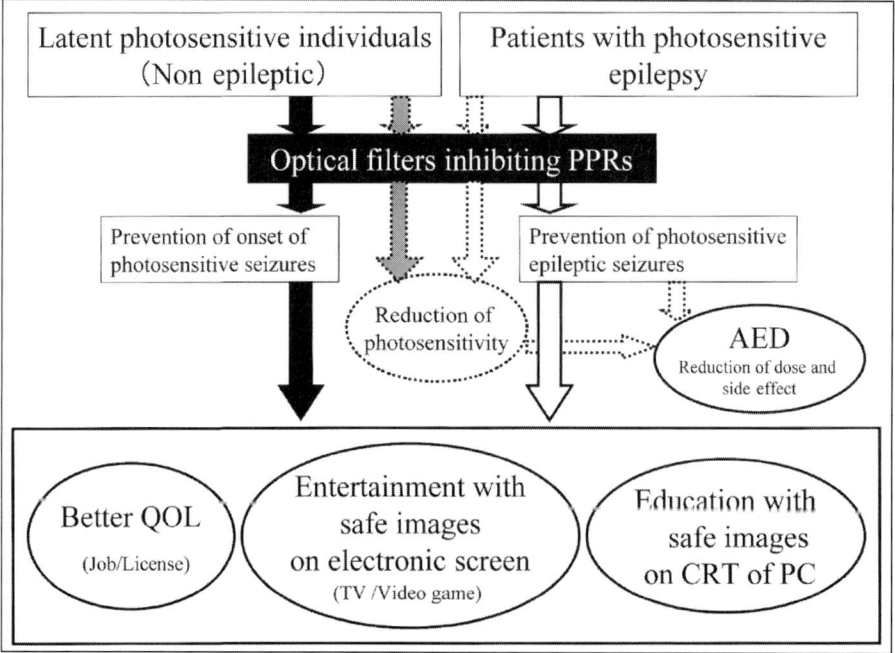

Figure 10. Effects of optical filters inhibiting PPRs in latent photosensitive nonepileptic patients and photosensitive epileptic patients. Dotted lines indicate probable effects. AED: antiepileptic drug; QOL: quality of life; CRT: cathode ray tube; PC: personal computer.

ameliorate the risk of seizures or epilepsy onset in persons with latent photosensitivity. In some epileptic patients, optical filters may make it possible to reduce the dosage of antiepileptic drugs and thus avoid their potential adverse effects. Moreover, the compound optical filters may have a unique role in the treatment of epileptic patients who have pure photosensitive seizures, that is, those who have no spontaneous seizures.

Finally, the use of personal computers for the education and amusement of children, who often have a high prevalence of photosensitivity, is spreading. Because the CRTs of personal computers are viewed at a closer distance than those of TV, the compound optical filters, by abolishing long-wavelength red light and reducing the quantity of emitted visible light, also have an important prophylactic potential in the use of personal computers.

Summary

Televised images are the most common stimulus for provoking photosensitive seizures in photosensitive persons. To inhibit photosensitive seizures in photosensitive persons who do or do not have epilepsy, we tried to develop innovative, nonpharmacological methods for reducing the levels of photic stimulation from televised images. Because the pathophysiological mechanisms for eliciting PPRs are both wavelength-dependent and quantity-of-light-dependent, we tested two different types of optical filters, one selectively reflecting long-wavelength red light, which stimulates the wavelength-dependent mechanism, and the other evenly absorbing light in the visible spectrum (neutral density filters). Each type of filter inhibited PPRs at an insufficient rate of less than 50%. Compound optical filters, composed of both types of filters, inhibited the PPRs at an adequate rate of approximately 90%. These compound optical filters cause few deviations of the chromaticity on emissions from the television's CRT. These filters might be useful as prophylactic tools against seizures induced by television viewing in photosensitive persons.

Acknowledgements

The authors thank Y. Kamiya and S. Murakami (Minolta) for spectroradiometry. This work was supported in part by Housou Bunka Foundation and Research Grants (13A-1 and 12B-2) for Nervous and Mental Disorders from the Ministry of Health and Welfare.

References

1. Binnie CD, Estevez O, Kasteleijn-Nolst Trenité DGA, Peters A. Colour and photosensitive epilepsy. *Electroencephalogr Clin Neurophysiol* 1984; 58: 387-91.
2. Binnie CD, Kasteleijn-Nolst Trenité DGA, De Korte R. Photosensitivity as a model for acute antiepileptic drug studies. *Electroencephalogr Clin Neurophysiol* 1986; 63: 35-41.

3. Binnie CD, Jeavons PM. Photosensitive epilepsies. In: Roger J, Bureau M, Dravet Ch, Dreifuss FE, Perret A, Wolf P, eds. *Epileptic syndromes in infancy, childhood and adolescence*. London: John Libbey, 1992; 299-305.
4. Buchthal F, Lennox M. The EEG effect of Metrazol and photic stimulation in 682 normal subjects. *Electroencephalogr Clin Neurophysiol* 1953; 5: 545-58.
5. Doose H, Waltz S. Photosensitivity: genetics and clinical significance. *Neuropediatrics* 1993; 24: 249-55.
6. Ebata K, Yagi K, Kamoshita S, Ushijima S, Miura H, Nishiura N, Mitsudome A. Report from survey group. In: Yamauchi T, ed. *Clinical study on photosensitive seizures*. Tokyo: Special Research Group of Ministry of Health and Welfare. 1998; 17-33.
7. Eeg-Olofsson O, Petersén I, Selden U. The development of the electroencephalogram in normal children from the age of 1 through 15 years. Paroxysmal activity. *Neuropädiatrie* 1971; 4: 375-404.
8. Furusho J, Sakanishi R, Tasaki I, Sato H, Yamaguchi K, Hoshi Y, Okabe T, Likura Y, Kumagai K. Background of "Pocket Monster" incident-questionnaire study in pediatric of emergency hospital. *No to Hattatsu* 1998; 30: 61-3.
9. Gregory RP, Oates T, Merry RTG. Electroencephalogram epileptiform abnormalities in candidates for aircrew training. *Electroencephalogr Clin Neurophysiol* 1993; 86: 75-7.
10. Harding GFA, Jeavons PM. *Photosensitive epilepsy. New edition*. London: MacKeith Press, 1994.
11. Harding GFA, Fylan F. Two visual mechanisms of photosensitivity. *Epilepsia* 1999; 40: 1446-51.
12. Klass DW, Fischer-Williams M. Sensory stimulation, sleep and sleep deprivation. In: *Handbook of electroencephalography and clinical neurophysiology, Vol. 3D*. Amsterdam: Elsevier, 1976; 5-73.
13. Kooi KA, Thomas MH, Mortenson FN. Photoconvulsive and photomyoclonic responses in adults. *Neurology* 1960; 10: 1051-8.
14. Mundy-Castle AC. Clinical significance of photic stimulation. *Electroencephalogr Clin Neurophysiol* 1953; 5: 187-202.
15. Takada H, Aso K, Watanabe K, Okumura A, Negoro T, Ishikawa T. Epileptic seizures induced by animated cartoon "Pocket Monster". *Epilepsia* 1999; 40: 997-1002.
16. Takahashi Y, Shigematsu H, Fujiwara T, Yagi K, Seino M. Self-induced photogenic seizures in a child with severe myoclonic epilepsy in infancy: optical investigations and treatments. *Epilepsia* 1995a; 36: 728-32.
17. Takahashi Y, Fujiwara T, Yagi K, Seino M. Wavelength specificity of photoparoxysmal responses in idiopathic generalised epilepsy. *Epilepsia* 1995b; 36: 1084-8.
18. Takahashi Y, Fujiwara T, Yagi K, Seino M. Wavelength dependency of photoparoxysmal responses in photosensitive nonepileptic subjects. *Tohoku J Exp Med* 1997a; 181: 311-9.
19. Takahashi Y, Watanabe M, Fujiwara T, Yagi K, Kondo N, Orii T, Seino M. Two different pathological conditions of photoparoxysmal responses in hereditary dentatorubral-pallidoluysian atrophy. *Brain Dev* 1997b; 19: 285-9.
20. Takahashi Y, Watanabe M, Ozawa T, Terasawa S, Motoyoshi F, Nakamura H, Yamada S, Okamoto H, Yamagishi A, Nakashima Y, Shimizu Y, Chikaishi T, Yajima S, Kondo N. Viewing condition of animated TV program called "Pocket Monsters" and induction of photosensitive seizures. *J Jpn Epilepsy Soc* 1999a; 17: 20-6.
21. Takahashi Y, Fujiwara T, Yagi K, Seino M. Photosensitive epilepsies and pathophysiological mechanisms of the photoparoxysmal response. *Neurology* 1999b; 53: 926-32.
22. Takahashi Y, Fujiwara T, Yagi K, Seino M. Wavelength dependency of photoparoxysmal responses in photosensitive epileptic patients. *Epilepsia* 1999c; 40 (suppl. 4): 23-7.
23. Takahashi Y, Ozawa T, Nakamura H, Yamada S, Okamoto H, Yajima S, Goto K, Kondo N. Long-wavelength red light emission from TV and photosensitive seizures. *Acta Neurol Scand* 2001; 103: 114-9.

Praxis induction and thinking induction: one or two mechanisms? A controversy

Y. Inoue*, B.G. Zifkin**

* National Epilepsy Center, Shizuoka Institute of Epilepsy and Neurological Disorders, Shizuoka, Japan
** Faculté de Médecine, Université de Montréal, Hôpital du Sacré-Cœur de Montréal; and Epilepsy Clinic, Montreal Neurological Hospital and Institute, Montreal, Quebec, Canada

▪ Introductory note (PW)

Over time, two separate traditions have developed in the epileptological literature about a particular part of the field of reflex epilepsies with complex precipitating mechanisms. The introduction of the term "praxis-induced seizures" was an attempt to develop a common perspective and understanding of cases that had been published under the most diverse terminologies, stretching from chess and card game epilepsy to seizures precipitated by decision-making. It is today widely accepted that these really belong in one group.

In parallel to this, another type of reflex epilepsy with seizures precipitated by thinking was proposed by other authors. This literature partially refers to the same cases as the above, and there are many similarities between the two concepts, which, however, are not identical.

Do we have to deal here with one or two distinct types of reflex epilepsy?

As both opinions are represented in the editorial board of this volume, it seemed a useful idea to have both positions represented in a controversy. This, however, took a somewhat unexpected turn. Dr. Inoue brings the discussion down to a point where the question remains how much of a difference it makes if a pathological response is already obtained when an action is thought of, or only when motor activity is added. As even in the case when no actual movement is involved, imaginations of spatial constructions seem to be at play. This could lead to the question whether spatial thinking, for a human, is possible at all without an inherent concept of moving in three-dimensional space.

Dr. Zifkin, however, moves one deliberate step further looking into the newly collected evidence of local cerebral activation with various steps of the cognitive and ideational processes involved here. We seem to be on a road of analysis where the controversy rapidly loses its importance as, on the background of these investigations, this problem can now be discussed on a level to which the meticulous description of the triggers was supposed to lead us later. Very appropriately, an analogy to Primary Reading Epilepsy (Wolf, 1994) is introduced where we have reached a similar level of understanding.

■ One mechanism (YI)

Introduction

Since the description of a patient with seizures induced by arithmetic tasks in 1962 (Ingvar & Nyman), an increasing number of similar cases of seizures precipitated by nonverbal, higher brain activities have been reported. The precipitation factors in these cases included arithmetics, writing, drawing, decision-making, playing cards, chess or other games, and thinking. As attempts to explain the mental processes involved in seizure induction, some hypotheses have been proposed, including the role of focusing attention (Ingvar & Nyman, 1962), complex and sequential decision-making (Forster, 1977), the importance of foreseeing the consequence of decision or strategic thinking (Cirignotta et al., 1980), the involvement of spatial processes (Wilkins et al., 1982), mathematical or spatial thinking (Goossens et al., 1990), and the importance of motor ideation or actual movement (Okazaki et al., 1981; Inoue et al., 1987; Matsuoka, 1989; Daniele et al., 1989; Yamamoto et al., 1991).

In a review of such cases reported under various terms in the literature, Inoue et al. (1994) indicated that the basic processes underlying the various precipitating factors share common features, and proposed to describe them by the term "praxis" (originally used by Daniele et al., 1989). The term implies that the seizures are precipitated when the patients are obliged to contemplate complicated spatial tasks in a sequential fashion, to make decisions, and to practically respond using a part of their body. The key step may be the transformation of thoughts into voluntary acts. Therefore, ideation of motor activity (or manipulation of spatial information underlying voluntary acts = spatial thinking) alone can induce a seizure, whereas simple handling can never be a trigger.

On the other hand, the term "induction by thinking" was preferred by some authors to designate probably the same patients (Andermann et al., 1998). Furthermore, some recent articles (Matsuoka et al., 2000; Zifkin & Andermann, 2001) considered thinking as a separate category from praxis.

Below, the concepts of praxis induction and thinking induction are summarized, and the similarities or possible differences between the two are discussed.

Praxis induction

The concept of praxis sensitivity has been described above. The precipitating factors include ideation or execution of complicated movements involving sequential spatial processing such as calculation, playing games, drawing, writing, construction, and complicated finger manipulations. Concentration of attention and stress are two important additional contributors to the precipitation of seizures.

A total of 92 patients with seizures induced by praxis were reported in 43 available publications. The clinical, EEG, and other characteristics of these patients are briefly summarized below (*for details see* Wolf & Inoue, 2002).

The sex distribution is 31 females and 61 males. For personal history, 57 of 84 patients with available information had no relevant events; while a history of febrile convulsion was reported in 16 patients, minor head injury in eight, meningitis/encephalopathy in three, and perinatal hypoxia in two. There was no neurological impairment in 83 of 84 patients. Intellectual function was documented in 60 patients, and often rated as average or above average.

The seizures usually started during adolescence at a mean age of 15 years. The seizures in these patients consisted of myoclonias in 78 patients, absences in 34, episodes of impairment of consciousness in two, other minor seizures in two, and generalised tonic-clonic seizures (GTC) in 80 patients. GTC either started suddenly or were preceded by a series of myoclonic jerks of increasing frequency.

Asymmetrical or focal features of the seizures were described in 25 patients; including myoclonias predominantly occurring in one hand in 18 patients, versive movement at seizure onset in eight patients, and focal seizure onset in two patients. Almost all patients had spontaneous seizures in addition to induced seizures.

The EEG presented interictal discharges of bilateral spikes, spike-waves or polyspike-waves in 54 of the 73 documented cases, with focal accentuation in seven and additional focal discharges in eight. Eighteen patients had no interictal paroxysmal activity. Twelve of 62 patients showed a photoparoxysmal response.

According to the clinical histories, the most frequently reported stimuli that evoked seizures were calculation in 42 patients, writing in 34, playing cards in 31, playing chess or similar games in 27, video games in 15, constructive activity in 12, drawing in 11, thinking (especially spatial thinking) in 10, decision-making in two, and additional complex finger manipulations in 19. In seven patients, playing musical instruments was also a trigger. Two patients had seizures triggered also by talking, two patients by reading, and two patients by eating. The seizures induced by talking and reading did not involve the arms but perioral muscles. In 58 patients, there was more than one effective trigger.

Reflex activation of paroxysmal EEG discharges by various neuropsychological tasks was confirmed in 82 patients, 15 of whom showed no epileptiform discharge in routine EEG. The evoked paroxysmal EEG discharges were almost the same as those recorded in the interictal state. Paroxysmal EEG activity could be induced by mental activity, which was previously not noticed by the individual patient.

Matsuoka *et al.* (2000) reported the results of EEG investigations with cognitive tasks, which they called neuropsychological EEG activation (NPA), in 480 patients with epilepsy. These tasks (reading, speaking, writing, written and mental arithmetic calculation, and spatial construction) provoked epileptic discharges in 38 patients (7.9%) and were accompanied by myoclonic seizures in 15 patients, absence seizures in eight, and simple partial seizures in one. The most effective trigger was writing (26 of 38 patients, 68.4%), followed by spatial construction (63.2%), written calculation (55.3%), mental calculation (7.9%), and reading (5.3%). The discharges evoked were quite similar to those that appeared spontaneously. They consisted of diffuse and symmetric spike-waves or polyspike-waves, but were sometimes concomitant with bilateral spike-waves that predominated over the central electrode site both with and without lateral asymmetry.

In summary, epilepsies with praxis-induced seizures have the following characteristics:

1. The precipitating stimuli involve both higher cortical and motor performances.

2. Seizures are typical of juvenile idiopathic generalised epilepsies with common unprovoked seizures.

3. Interictal and ictal EEG almost always consist of bilateral, mostly symmetric runs of spike-waves.

Induction by thinking

The term "thinking induction" was coined by Wilkins *et al.* (1982). They described a 45-year-old patient with absences, myoclonias and GTCs since age 12 years. The seizures were induced by card games, calculation, mental arithmetic, and puzzles. Drawing, letter outline, mental control and arithmetics, especially mental multiplication or division induced paroxysmal activity under testing conditions. They emphasized the role of manipulation of spatial information in EEG induction, and speculated that this type of thought activates the parietal lobe before inducing electroencephalographic or clinical seizures, because mental arithmetic also involves spatial processing. The same opinion was expressed by Andermann *et al.* (1989, 1998) and by Goossens *et al.* (1990).

Andermann *et al.* (1998) reviewed the clinical features of epilepsy induced by thinking and spatial tasks in nine cases of their own and an additional 16 cases reported in the literature. The most frequently reported stimuli that provoked seizures were playing cards in 15 patients, calculation in 14, playing chess in 11, and playing checkers in five. Other stimuli such as measuring or drawing complex figures were less frequently reported. These precipitating factors are apparently not much different from those observed in praxis induction. Other clinical and EEG features were quite similar to those reported for praxis induction, mainly because there was an overlapping of patients in both studies.

In the study of Matsuoka *et al.* (2000), patients were initially examined by routine reading, speaking, calculation, writing and spatial construction tasks; and when EEG paroxysms were activated, they were examined by more detailed NPA that included mental sentence construction, visualizing letters, mental calculation and mental spatial construction. The results of the 38 patients showed that EEG paroxysms were always induced by higher mental activities requiring hand movements (action-programming type) in 32 patients. In four patients they were induced by both mental activities requiring hand movements and activities not accompanied by hand movements (thinking type). No EEG paroxysm was induced by motor activity alone.

For the four patients with thinking type precipitation, the triggers other than thinking were drawing, constructive acts, written calculation and writing. These are not categorically different from the triggers in the action-programming type.

Andermann et al. (1998) pointed out that the condition described as praxis induction emphasizes the role of a motor component in the activity process. According to their experience, the requirement for hand movements before activation is rare. However, as already mentioned, praxis involves ideation of motor activity and is not necessarily accompanied by actual movement. Spatial processing (manipulation of space) is strongly associated with the representation of movements. Thus the distinction of thinking type and "nonthinking" type (or action-programming type of Matsuoka et al.) precipitations according to the presence or absence of actual movements seems not practical. This point will be further discussed below.

Praxis induction vs. thinking induction

In order to scrutinize the possible differences between praxis induction and thinking induction, we compared 20 cases in which "thinking" or purely mental activities were explicitly reported as precipitating factors with 74 cases in which "thinking" was not mentioned as a precipitator. In most cases of the former group, thinking was not the only trigger; calculation, writing, construction or hand movement also induced seizures.

These two groups of patients shared quite similar clinical and electrographic characteristics. Only slight differences were found in family history of seizures and photosensitivity, but they were not significant (Table I).

The precipitating factors other than thinking were also quite similar. Only slight differences were found in playing cards and writing, with a slightly higher frequency in the "nonthinking" group (Table II).

Thus, there is no evidence of a significant difference between praxis induction and thinking induction. This result is consistent with the findings of Inoue et al. (1992) who performed a cluster analysis of the precipitating factors in 74 cases. They revealed three relative independent groups: calculation and playing chess; drawing, writing and spatial tasks; and playing cards and finger manipulations. Spatial tasks including thinking did not constitute a distinct group.

However, there were two reports indicating that absences or bland spells were more often induced by abstract thinking such as spatial tasks or mental calculation, while myoclonias were often precipitated by activities accompanying actual hand or finger movements (Ohtaka et al., 1977; Yamamoto et al., 1990).

Table I. Seizure induction by thinking vs. nonthinking (1): Clinical features

	Precipitated by thinking	Not precipitated by thinking
N	20	74
M/F	16/4	45/29
Past history	4/18 (22%)	25/68 (37%)
Family history	2/18 (11%)	22/66 (33%)
Age of onset (yr)	14.8	15.3
Myoclonia	16 (80%)	62 (84%)
Absences	6 (30%)	27 (36%)
Convulsions	17 (85%)	65 (88%)
Focal features	5 (25%)	20 (27%)
Photosensitivity	1/13 (8%)	11/51 (22%)

Table II. Seizure induction by thinking vs. nonthinking (2): Precipitation factors other than thinking

Other precipitating factors	Precipitated by thinking	Not precipitated by thinking
Chess	6 (30%)	20 (27%)
Card	4 (20%)	35 (47%)
Games	3 (15%)	6 (8%)
Drawing	5 (25%)	19 (26%)
Construction	10 (50%)	26 (35%)
Mathematics	15 (75%)	47 (64%)
Writing	5 (25%)	36 (49%)
Manipulation	4 (20%)	15 (20%)

Ohtaka et al. (1977) described a 35-year-old male patient with a history of birth asphyxia and three episodes of febrile convulsion. GTC occurred at 14 years of age. Since age 20, he noticed myoclonias of the hand when writing Kanji, i.e. Japanese ideographic script. Myoclonias of the jaw were observed when reading complex sentences aloud. There was clouding of consciousness when mentally constructing a complex sentence. No EEG information was available.

Yamamoto et al. (1990) reported a 31-year-old female patient with myoclonias induced by fine finger movement and calculation using abacus since 17 years of age. At age 18, a GTC occurred during a mathematical examination. Myoclonias, absences and GTC were induced by calculation, sewing, cooking or copying. At examination, EEG paroxysms were most often provoked by mental arithmetics and calculation using abacus. Calculation with an abacus induced myoclonias of the hand being used, and mental arithmetics induced absences without myoclonias, although the EEG paroxysms induced in both occasions were quite similar.

These anecdotal observations are very interesting in that they suggest that the clinical manifestations induced may differ depending on the nature of precipitation, although this hypothesis could not be confirmed in the above comparative clinical study. One could well speculate that the seizures differ depending on the cortical areas or generalising processes activated, and spatial thinking and actual movement may represent the two extremes of a continuum of precipitation mechanisms.

Our own experience of two patients would be worth mentioning here. The first patient (a 35-year-old male patient with myoclonias, absences and GTC since 12 years of age) had a documented episode of absence with mild myoclonias when he was using or about to use the fingers to construct block designs, but the same patient had absences without myoclonias when he was thinking without finger movements in the same test session. The ictal EEG was quite similar in both occasions (bilateral diffuse spike-waves).

The second patient (a 23-year-old male patient with myoclonias, absences and GTC since 12 years of age) also had myoclonias induced by constructing block design. Myoclonias or myoclonias followed by absence were induced by constructing with finger movements. However, similar seizures, although somewhat milder, were also induced when he did not move his fingers. There was no difference in the ictal EEG (bilateral diffuse polyspikes followed by spike-waves).

Thus, the hypothesis that the clinical manifestations induced differ depending on the involvement of functional anatomic areas activated by a variety of precipitating mechanisms would be supported by the first case but not by the second. The presence or absence of actual motor activity may not be important in praxis induction, because motor activity is already represented in the precipitation regardless of the execution of actual movement. It is also possible that clinical seizure observation may not be sensitive enough to differentiate the spectrum of precipitation.

The term "thinking" has a broad meaning, including not only spatial but also emotional and linguistic aspects. But, if limited to spatial thinking, thinking induction may be almost identical to praxis induction, because spatial thinking almost always involves representation of movement.

Summary

The fundamental mechanism of praxis induction is nonverbal sequential spatial processing that induces clinical manifestations of myoclonias or absences. Praxis is not necessarily accompanied by actual movement, but includes ideation of motor activity (or manipulation of spatial information = spatial thinking). Therefore, spatial thinking alone can induce a seizure.

The concept of thinking induction is covered by the definition of praxis induction. Therefore, praxis induction seems to be a more appropriate term to express the spectrum of seizure induction by nonverbal higher brain function.

Two mechanisms (BZ)

Introduction

We will take the position that seizures induced by thinking and praxis-induced seizures involve two different mechanisms and that these can be distinguished based on clinical and experimental evidence. We will first review the history of these two entities and then discuss what these mechanisms may be, how they are similar, and how they are different. Reflex seizures induced by such cognitive tasks have been regarded as a rarity and have not been studied extensively in Europe or in North America; interest in "praxis induction" has been largely found in Japan. This may reflect a disproportionate interest in medically intractable symptomatic and cryptogenic epilepsy in North American epilepsy centres, which are usually focused on epilepsy surgery: patients with idiopathic generalised epilepsy are usually more responsive to antiepileptic drugs and may be less likely to be evaluated by academic epilepsy specialists.

Seizures induced by thinking

First described by Ingvar and Nyman (1962) as "epilepsia arithmetices" in a patient whose seizures were induced by calculation, the term "seizures induced by thinking" was introduced by Wilkins et al. (1982). This more general term was used because review of cases reported to that time, later expanded by Goossens et al. (1990) and by Andermann et al. (1998), showed that patients reporting seizures triggered by mental arithmetic, almost all with an idiopathic generalised epilepsy (IGE), were also triggered by nonarithmetic cognitive tasks, and because other patients with seizures activated by other nonverbal cognitive tasks had a similar clinical and EEG pattern to those reporting activation by arithmetic. Many complex mental activities have been reported to trigger seizures, such as card games and board games such as checkers, or making complex decisions. But interestingly, these seizures do not typically appear to be activated by reading, writing, or by explicitly verbal tasks. Most patients have more than one seizure trigger identified either by history or by EEG monitoring with neuropsychological testing. Seizures can be triggered in at least some of these patients without any real or contemplated movement of the hands (*e.g.* by a task requiring a spoken answer to an orally presented arithmetic or spatial problem). Patients usually appear to have spontaneous seizures also, and almost all reported patients have had generalised convulsions. Often these begin after a period of myoclonic jerks, but myoclonic jerks occurred without a following convulsion in 76% of patients described by Andermann et al. (1998) and 60% of patients had absence seizures often associated with myoclonic jerks. Pure absence epilepsy with seizures triggered by thinking was not seen, but not all patients had myoclonus although some probably had juvenile myoclonic epilepsy (JME). Myoclonic jerks and absence attacks may be ignored or unreported until a generalised seizure occurs and the patient then comes to medical attention. Clinical and EEG responses to triggers and the interictal EEG abnormalities may all be modified or abolished by antiepileptic drugs especially valproate, and reports of such patients must be cautiously interpreted.

Praxis-induced seizures

Praxis induction involves seizures triggered by thinking about "complicated spatial tasks in a sequential fashion, decisions, and practically responding by using a part of the body" (Inoue, 2001). Writing is reported to be a major precipitating factor (Inoue et al., 1994). Simple repetitive hand or finger movements without "action-programming activity" (defined as "higher mental activity requiring hand movement" and apparently synonymous with praxis) are not effective triggers, and patients do not appear to have reading epilepsy (Matsuoka et al., 2000). Praxis induction seems closely linked to myoclonus as part of both triggered and apparently spontaneous attacks and is found almost exclusively in JME. It does not seem prominent in patients with thinking-induced seizures who do not also have prominent myoclonic reflex attacks. In its milder or most restricted forms, such as the morning myoclonic jerk of the arm manipulating a utensil (Seino M, personal communication, Bethel-Bielefeld, 1999), this phenomenon resembles cortical reflex myoclonus as part of a "continuum of epileptic activity centered on the sensorimotor cortex" (Vignal et al., 1998). The motor component, either imagined or performed, is crucial in praxis induction but many other patients with seizures induced by thinking are activated by tasks such as purely mental calculation of orally presented arithmetic tasks with no motor component in either the stimulus or the spoken response.

Important similarities and differences

An important common factor in these two clinical entities is that "thinking" in a nonverbal way seems to be an essential element of the trigger for both, especially as even those activated by action are not sensitive to mere proprioceptive stimulation or repetitive finger movement. They have to "think" also if a seizure is to be triggered.

An important clinical difference is that in seizures induced by thinking, this motor component is not necessary to trigger seizures. We shall attempt to show that this difference can be related to different mechanisms of seizure triggering.

Pathophysiology of reflex seizures with underlying idiopathic generalised epilepsy

Clementi (1929) induced focal seizures with photic stimulation in dogs after applying strychnine to the occipital cortex to make it hyperexcitable. He also showed that seizures could be triggered even if only a limited area was treated with strychnine as long as it was applied to both occipital cortices. Recruitment of a "critical mass" of epileptogenic cortex in response to the reflex seizure stimulus can result in epileptiform EEG activity or a clinical seizure. This recruitment can be understood as relatively direct in some, but in other cases may involve the participation and interaction of several cortical areas or of cortex and subcortical structures activated by the external trigger. Considering the model of a chronic epileptic focus (Wyler & Ward, 1980), Wieser proposes that epileptogenic stimuli produce temporary recruitment of Group 2 epileptic neurons into the effective quantity of epileptic cortex to reach a critical mass (Wieser, 1998).

Seizures induced by thinking occur in patients with idiopathic generalised epilepsy despite the regional or functional nature of the trigger. The clinical and EEG syndrome of a functional trigger eliciting generalised events was first well documented with pattern-sensitivity and later in many cases of primary reading epilepsy.

In pattern-sensitive subjects, generalised seizures can occur if normal excitation of visual cortex involves a "critical mass" of cortical area with synchronization and subsequent spreading of excitation from the occipital cortex trigger (Binnie et al., 1985). The model of human pattern-sensitive epilepsy is of special interest because it shows that generalised clinical events and EEG abnormalities can be activated by a specific functional stimulation with a known localization (reviewed by Binnie & Wilkins, 1998), a electroclinical syndrome which is found in many subjects with reflex seizures and IGE, and who are thus presumed to have diffuse cortical hyperexcitability. Photosensitive occipital partial seizures also occur in patients with IGE, and motor activity can elicit seizures in nearly 50% of patients with JME (Matsuoka et al., 2000). These and other observations in both reflex and spontaneous epileptogenesis (reviewed by Binnie, this volume) suggest that the postulated cortical hyperexcitability in IGE is not necessarily uniform: specific activities can activate specific cortical systems and produce focal discharges or partial seizures, which may generalise. This does not invalidate a diagnosis of underlying generalised epilepsy but shows that the biological substrate of generalised epilepsy can be complicated.

In a patient with idiopathic generalised epilepsy and seizures induced by thinking, Wilkins and associates documented the increased likelihood of thinking-induced paroxysmal EEG activity with increasing task difficulty. They suggested that increasing difficulty of parietal lobe and possibly frontal lobe epileptogenic stimuli led to increasing regional recruitment to reach a critical mass of epileptogenic cortex with activation of generalised epileptiform activity, analogous to the activation of such generalised activity by the occipital cortical activation produced by the stimuli of pattern sensitive epilepsy (Wilkins et al., 1982).

Models for seizures induced by thinking and by "praxis"?

New information obtained by functional MRI (fMRI) and evoked potential studies shows that number processing is associated with a specific cerebral network in the inferior intraparietal area of *both* hemispheres and that activation of this network is not dependent on hand or eye movement or task difficulty. There is, however, regional specialization and lateralization within this network: exact arithmetic shows preferential fMRI activation over various left (dominant) hemisphere regions especially in the parietal lobe, but larger or more difficult problems cause activation of the same bilateral parietal areas as does approximate arithmetic, which shows language independence (Dehaene et al., 1999). Importantly, these data suggest that only the (dominant hemisphere) verbal circuit is used for well-rehearsed exact arithmetic facts such as the multiplication table. One would thus expect dissociations in patients with lesional acquired dyscalculia, which is in fact observed (Stanescu-Cosson et al., 2000). In the light of this, we recently reviewed detailed results in a subject with seizures induced by thinking (originally reported in Wilkins et al., 1982), whose EEG abnormalities could not be triggered by single-digit multiplication but who was readily triggered by division with remainder or by more complex multiplication tasks (in retrospect, probably involving approximate arithmetic), suggesting that unilateral dominant parietal activation was inadequate to trigger seizures and that bilateral activation of this network was required to induce seizures with arithmetic tasks in this patient. During monitoring, seizures could be triggered by orally presented tasks with no motor components. Triggered seizures were brief absence attacks without polyspike EEG activity or myoclonus and he also reported generalised convulsions without myoclonus triggered by mental arithmetic in daily life. Monitoring showed that episodes of limb shaking were anxiety attacks and not myoclonus. He was not taking valproate. Thus there was no evidence for praxis as an essential element in triggering his seizures, and he did not appear to have JME. Similarly, some of the subjects in Matsuoka's detailed study (2000) were activated without "action programming" and were classified as having seizures induced by thinking.

Models of the structures involved with induction of seizures by thinking and action combined may be provided by fMRI and EP study of a number comparison task with a motor response by one hand. These methods break the task into steps: visual identification, magnitude comparison, and response elaboration and execution. These steps are found to successively activate the right fusiform gyrus, bilateral parietal structures; and *for the motor response only*, the sensorimotor, supplementary motor, and insular cortices contralateral to the responding hand (Pinel *et al.*, 1999). One may then surmise that praxis induction, which is more than simple seizure triggering by proprioceptive input or by simple repetitive movement, must involve more widespread cerebral areas than those which are sufficient for seizure triggering by arithmetic or spatial problems without motor responses. Praxis induction must activate a critical mass of hyperexcitable cortex beyond parietal cortices and beyond the network subsuming spatial thought. In particular, such tasks must activate the sensorimotor areas, which are also preferentially involved in JME, with which praxis induction is strongly associated. Matsuoka (2000) notes that "it is likely that IGE seizures induced by higher mental activity consist of at least two forms: seizures induced by thinking and spatial tasks, and seizures induced by writing, written calculation or drawing requiring action-programming activity. These two forms would either show distinct mechanisms of seizure induction or represent two ends of a pathophysiological continuum".

In both cases, it appears that "thinking" in a nonverbal way seems to be the essential triggering element, especially as patients activated by praxis are not sensitive to mere proprioceptive stimulation. Inoue *et al.* (1994), have aptly summarized this as nonlesional reflex epilepsy evoked by nonlinguistic higher cerebral activities.

The close relation of praxis induction to JME should be considered. Similar to occipital triggering in pattern sensitivity, one can argue that praxis induction depends on enhanced functional or regional hyperexcitability in the Rolandic areas in addition to any other regional or network hyperexcitability that may be present. Regional hyperexcitability also seems to be a feature of JME: clinically, the spontaneous myoclonus may be asymmetric or prolonged without a following generalised convulsion or alteration of awareness, and versive seizures can also occur. Similarly, the praxis-induced seizures, myoclonic attacks mainly involving initially the arm and hand, often do not generalise and remain as essentially regional motor events without tonic-clonic seizures or evident impairment of consciousness. The EEG is also not homogeneously disturbed in JME and the triggered and spontaneous ictal epileptiform abnormalities are quite similar. Scalp EEG showed focal interictal discharges in 30.3% of JME patients studied in detail in one study by Panayiotopoulos et al. (1994) and focal EEG abnormalities of all kinds in 36.7% (Aliberti et al., 1994). Panayiotopoulos also commented on the precipitation of seizures by mental activation and other factors as part of the syndrome. Wolf (1994) emphasized the typical frontocentral predominance of the ictal EEG activity recorded with the myoclonic jerks of JME. This asymmetry has been discussed by several authors (reviewed by Matsuoka et al., 2000). Berkovic (1994) interpreted regional predominance of the spike and wave activity of IGE as implying involvement of specific corticothalamic loops, reminiscent of the "*secteurs aréo-thalamiques*" proposed by Gastaut (1950), and suggested that reflex triggers in these patients represent specific local mechanisms that entrain these loops. Woermann et al. (1998), have shown that quantitative MRI suggests differences in patients with myoclonus who also have JME and note that such "... structural cortical changes may be associated with abnormalities in functional connectivity". Further studies in patients with JME have shown abnormalities in mesial frontal structures in many (Woermann et al., 1999): it would be of interest to find whether subjects with these findings are more prone to reflex activation.

One mechanism or two?

The degree to which one may defend the idea of two separate mechanisms depends on the level of detail at which the distinction is to be made, and this is admittedly arbitrary. There are lumpers and splitters and each approach within reason has its uses. There appear to be some common characteristics among patients with IGE and reflex seizures of different types as discussed above, in which a trigger activating a functional network induces clinically and electroencephalographically generalised or at least bilateral seizures. These observations have led to useful discussion of the nature of generalised epilepsy, but clear distinctions are possible and necessary between, for example, reading epilepsy and pattern-sensitive epilepsy despite the undeniably shared basic features. Only scanty and inconclusive pathological information is available for human IGE in the decades since these reflex seizures were first studied, but information is recently available from techniques enabling at least an approximate mapping of both cognitive and executive brain processes and very detailed morphologic imaging. It is thus perhaps less useful now to take too broad a view of reflex epileptogenesis, especially in IGE, and especially not for all IGE syndromes.

Thus we suggest that two mechanisms can be identified for seizures induced by thinking and praxis-induced seizures. In the first, nonverbal activation of a biparietal network seems necessary and sufficient for seizure triggering in predisposed individuals, without excluding more extensive activation in some patients and by some stimuli: motor activation is neither necessary nor sufficient for these events.

A second mechanism is proposed for praxis induction. Praxis induction requires actual or contemplated movements, and is particularly associated with JME. The impulses to trigger these seizures, wherever their origin, must eventually gain access to sensorimotor areas and then activate them: these regions must be preferentially hyperexcitable and perhaps abnormally linked to other areas to constitute the critical mass needed for seizure induction. This may involve corticocortical paths to the hyperexcitable cortex, similar to the activation of hyperexcitable frontorolandic cortex by non-hyperexcitable visual afferents in simian photosensitivity. This particular sensorimotor regional or functional hyperexcitability is neither necessary nor sufficient in seizures induced by thinking but appears necessary in praxis induction. This pattern fits well with JME, in which there is apparent regional hyperexcitability of sensorimotor cortex and possibly relevant morphologic abnormalities involving the motor system as well.

References

1. Aliberti V, Grunewald RA, Panayiotopoulos CP, Chroni E. Focal electroencephalographic abnormalities in juvenile myoclonic epilepsy. *Epilepsia* 1994; 35: 297-301.
2. Andermann F, Goossens L, Andermann E. Clinical features and diagnosis of epilepsy induced by thinking. In: Beaumanoir A, Gastaut H, Naquet R, eds. *Reflex seizures and reflex epilepsies*. Geneva: Médecine & Hygiène, 1989; 317-22.
3. Andermann F, Zifkin BG, Andermann E. Epilepsy induced by thinking and spatial tasks. In: Zifkin BG, Andermann F, Beaumanoir A, Rowan AJ, eds. *Reflex epilepsies and reflex seizures. Advances in Neurology*, vol. 75. Philadelphia: Lippincott-Raven, 1998; 263-72.
4. Berkovic S. Regional manifestations of idiopathic epilepsy: an antithesis. In: Wolf P, ed. *Epileptic seizures and syndromes*. London: John Libbey; 1994: 267-8.
5. Binnie CD, Findlay J, Wilkins AJ. Mechanisms of epileptogenesis in photosensitive epilepsy implied by the effects of moving patterns. *Electroencephalogr Clin Neurophysiol* 1985; 61: 1-6.
6. Binnie CD, Wilkins AJ. Visually Induced seizures not caused by flicker (intermittent light stimulation). In: Zifkin BG, Andermann F, Beaumanoir A, Rowan AJ, eds. *Reflex epilepsies and reflex seizures. Advances in Neurology*, vol. 75. Philadelphia: Lippincott-Raven Press, 1998: 123-38.
7. Cirignotta R, Cicogna P, Lugaresi E. Epileptic seizures during card games and draughts. *Epilepsia* 1980; 21: 137-40.
8. Clementi A. Stricninizzazione della sfera corticale visiva ed epilessia sperimentale da stimoli luminosi. *Arch Fisiol* 1929; 27: 356-87.
9. Daniele O, Raieli V, Mattaliano A, Natale E. Seizures precipitated by unusual epileptogenic tasks. In: Beaumanoir A, Gastaut H, Naquet R, eds. *Reflex seizures and reflex epilepsies*. Geneva: Médecine & Hygiène, 1989; 333-6.
10. Dehaene S, Spelke E, Pinel P, Stanescu R, Tsivkin S. Sources of mathematical thinking: Behavioral and brain-imaging evidence. *Science* 1999; 284: 970-4.
11. Forster FM. *Reflex epilepsy, behavioral therapy and conditional reflexes*. Springfield: Thomas, 1977; 94-134.
12. Gastaut H. Évidences électrographiques d'un mécanisme sous-cortical dans certaines épilepsies partielles – La signification clinique des secteurs "aréothalamiques". *Revue Neurologique* 1950; 83: 396-401.
13. Goossens L, Andermann F, Andermann E, Remillard GM. Reflex seizures induced by calculation, card or board games, and spatial tasks: a review of 25 patients and delineation of the epileptic syndromes. *Neurology* 1990; 40: 1171-6.
14. Ingvar DH, Nyman GE. Epilepsia arithmetices: a new psychologic trigger mechanism in a case of epilepsy. *Neurology* 1962; 12: 282-7.

15. Inoue Y, Seino M, Tanaka M, Kubota H, Yamakaku K, Yagi K. Epilepsy with praxis-induced seizures. In: Wolf P, ed. *Epileptic seizures and syndromes*. London: John Libbey, 1994; 81-91.
16. Inoue Y, Yagi K, Muramatsu R, Morikawa T, Tottori T, Seino M. Three cases of reflex epilepsy evoked by nonlinguistic higher cerebral activities. *J Jpn Epil Soc* 1987; 5: 106-14.
17. Inoue Y, Suzuki S, Watanabe Y, Yagi K, Seino M. Nonlesional reflex epilepsy evoked by nonverbal higher cerebral activities. *J Jpn Epil Soc* 1992; 10: 1-9.
18. Matsuoka H. A clinical and electroencephalographic study of juvenile myoclonic epilepsy: its pathophysiological considerations based on the findings obtained from neuropsychological EEG activation. *Psychiatr Neurol* (Japan) 1989; 91: 318-46.
19. Matsuoka H, Takahashi T, Sasaki M, Matsumoto K, Yoshida S, Numachi Y, Saito H, Ueno T, Sato M. Neuropsychological EEG activation in patients with epilepsy. *Brain* 2000; 123, 318-30.
20. Ohtaka T, Miyasaka M. A case of language-induced epilepsy precipitated mainly by writing. *Psychiatry Neurol* (Japan) 1977; 79: 587-601.
21. Okazaki K, Kato N, Toshida S, Fukuyama Y, Kazamatsuri H. Reflex epilepsy evoked by fine movements of upper limbs and accompanying stressful situation: report of two cases. *Psychiatry* (Japan) 1981; 23: 1241-9.
22. Panayiotopoulos CP, Obeid T, Tahan AR. Juvenile myoclonic epilepsy: a 5-year prospective study. *Epilepsia* 1994; 35: 285-96.
23. Pinel P, Le Clec'h G, van de Moortele PF, Naccache L, Le Bihan D, Dehaene S. Event-related fMRI analysis of the cerebral circuit for number comparison. *Neuroreport* 1999; 10: 1473-9.
24. Stanescu-Cosson R, Pinel P, van de Moortele PF, Le Bihan D, Cohen L, Dehaene S. Understanding dissociations in dyscalculia: a brain imaging study of the impact of number size on the cerebral networks for exact and approximate calculation. *Brain* 2000; 123: 2240-55.
25. Vignal JP, Biraben A, Chauvel PY, Reutens DC. Reflex partial seizures of sensorimotor cortex (including cortical reflex myoclonus and startle epilepsy). In: Zifkin BG, Andermann F, Beaumanoir A, Rowan AJ, eds. *Reflex epilepsies and reflex seizures. Advances in Neurology, vol. 75*. Philadelphia: Lippincott-Raven, 1998; 207-26.
26. Wieser HG. Seizure induction in reflex seizures and reflex epilepsy. In: Zifkin BG, Andermann F, Beaumanoir A, Rowan AJ, eds. *Reflex epilepsies and reflex seizures. Advances in Neurology, vol. 75*. Philadelphia: Lippincott-Raven, 1998; 69-85.
27. Wilkins A, Zifkin B, Andermann F, McGovern E. Seizures induced by thinking. *Ann Neurol* 1982; 11: 608-12.
28. Woermann FG, Sisodiya SM, Free SL, Duncan JS. Quantitative MRI in patients with idiopathic generalised epilepsy. Evidence of widespread cerebral structural changes. *Brain* 1998; 121: 1661-7.
29. Woermann FG, Free SL, Koepp MJ, Sisodiya SM, Duncan JS. Abnormal cerebral structure in juvenile myoclonic epilepsy demonstrated with voxel-based analysis of MRI. *Brain* 1999; 122: 2111-8.
30. Wolf P. Regional manifestation of idiopathic epilepsy. Introduction. In: Wolf P, ed. *Epileptic seizures and syndromes*. London: John Libbey, 1994; 265-7.
31. Wolf P. Reading epilepsy. In: Wolf P, ed. *Epileptic Seizures and Syndromes, With Some of their Theoretical Implications*. London: John Libbey, 1994; 67-73.
32. Wolf P, Inoue Y. Complex reflex epilepsies: reading epilepsy and praxis-induction. In: Roger J, Bureau M, Dravet Ch, Tassinari CA, Wolf P, eds. *Epileptic syndromes in infancy, childhood and adolescence. 3rd edition*. Eastleigh: John Libbey, 2002; 315-25.
33. Wyler AR, Ward AA Jr. Epileptic neurons. In: Lockard JS, Ward AA Jr, eds. *Epilepsy. A Window to Brain Mechanisms*. New York: Raven Press, 1980; 51-68.
34. Yamamoto S, Egawa I, Yamamoto J, Kawasaki T, Yamashita K, Shiraishi J, Shimizu A. A case of reflex epilepsy induced by higher mental activities, mainly by arithmetics. *J Jpn Epil Soc* 1990; 8: 22-8.

35. Yamamoto J, Egawa I, Yamamoto S, Shimizu A. Reflex epilepsy induced by calculation using a "soroban", a Japanese traditional calculator. *Epilepsia* 1991; 32: 39-43.
36. Zifkin B, Andermann F. Epilepsy with reflex seizures. In: Wyllie E, ed. *The treatment of epilepsy (3rd edition)*. Philadelphia: Lippincott Williams & Wilkins, 2001; 537-49.

Perioral reflex myoclonias in reading epilepsy and juvenile myoclonic epilepsy

T. Mayer, P. Wolf

Danish Epilepsy Centre Dianalund, Dianalund, Denmark

Introduction

Reading epilepsy (RE) is a rare syndrome with a male preponderance and a strong genetic component (Wolf, 1992; Mayer & Wolf, 1999). According to the International Classification of Epilepsies and Epileptic Syndromes "all or almost all seizures in the syndrome of RE are precipitated by reading (especially aloud) and are independent of the content of the text. They are simple focal motor-involving masticatory muscles, or visual, and if the stimulus is not interrupted, generalised tonic-clonic seizures (GTCS) may occur". Seizures usually start in late puberty; the course is benign with little tendency to spontaneous seizures. Physical examination and imaging studies are normal.

The seizures in RE are myoclonic, seldom tonic or tonic-clonic seizures; the consciousness is clear in myoclonic or tonic seizures. The main seizure type is myoclonic, involving the perioral muscles, triggered by reading (aloud and silently); in 25%-30% of the patients also talking. This was long considered a more or less exclusive seizure type for this syndrome (Wolf, 1992). However, since we became aware of the frequency of identical myoclonias in juvenile myoclonic epilepsy (JME), where they are triggered by talking and less frequently by reading (Mayer & Wolf, 1997, 1999), we prefer to call these myoclonias which don't occur spontaneously, perioral reflex myoclonias (PORM) (Wolf & Mayer, 2000). PORM are short, sometimes repetitive, abrupt myoclonia around the mouth which will clearly be noticed by the patients, sometimes with interruption of reading and speaking. Most of these jerks appear strongly localized and do not change the side in individual patients. In some cases, PORM are bilateral. We defined PORM with associated symptoms (*e.g.* eyelid myoclonia) as PORM plus.

PORM are the leading symptom in RE. Sometimes they appear in variants such as:

- Abnormal sensations or non-myoclonic movements in the muscles which are involved in reading and talking (tongue, throat, jaw, lips, face).
- Sensations in parts of the face which are involved in talking and reading, like stiffness, numbness, tightness, clicking sensations, and stammering.

In his early paper, Bickford (1956) distinguished primary and secondary RE. The primary form, in which only reading-induced seizures occur, belongs to the idiopathic localisation-related epilepsy syndromes. Secondary reading epilepsies, in which spontaneous and reading-induced seizures (e.g. psychomotor seizures) occur, belong to different epilepsy syndromes (e.g. symptomatic focal epilepsies). There is an ongoing controversial discussion about this classification; especially the term "secondary" can be misunderstood. One proposal, made by Bickford himself (1973), was to distinguish a specific (= "primary") form from a nonspecific (= "secondary") form. The idea behind this was to distinguish a genetic syndrome (the primary form) from other forms, where reading-induced seizures are part of complex syndromes including spontaneous seizures. Since Radhakrishan and co-workers (1995) and also our group (Mayer & Wolf, 1997) published several patients with what seemed to be a co-occurrence (Radhakrishan et al., 1995) of RE and JME, there is also a discussion whether RE should be considered an idiopathic generalised epilepsy syndrome.

EEG findings in RE

In the routine EEG, nearly 80% of the findings are negative (Wolf, 1992). Infrequently, bilateral spike and waves or temporal sharp waves are seen. Photic stimulation is positive in about only 10% of the cases (Wolf, 1992). Ictal findings are variable and unimpressive. Paroxysmal discharges were found in 76.8% of the investigations, 30.1% of them focal, 38.4% bilateral but lateralized, and 31.5% bilateral symmetric. If there is a localised discharge, in 75% of the cases it is temporal, in 25% of the cases frontal. There is a left predominance of 78% of the cases with a localised discharge (Wolf, 1992).

Pathophysiology of PORM

The clinical symptoms of PORM bear the characteristics of cortical reflex myoclonias (CRM): the CRM is related to a small area of the sensorimotor cortex; it typically involves only a few adjacent muscles (Hallett, 1985).

The common precipitating mechanism in RE is the pivotal formal act in reading, i.e. the transformation of graphemes into phonemes (Wolf, 1992). In patients with RE, the sensorimotor cortex is not hyperexcitable per se, because spontaneous seizures never occur. A hypothesis exists that the hyperexcitable neuronal network that subserves speech may drive the relative motor cortex effectively through a direct transcortical pathway (Hallett, 1979; Obeso et al., 1985). This assumed bilaterally hyperexcitable speech network, under reading provocation, would give rise to bilateral myoclonic jerks, which need not be necessarily symmetric (Koutroumanidis et al., 1998). Bartolomei and co-workers (1999) reported on findings of back-averaging in a 53-year-old patient who had experienced isolated myoclonias of the right face for more than ten years, induced by talking, reading and writing. She also had Morbus Parkinson, treated with L-Dopa and suffered from Diabetes mellitus. In the MRT imaging a slight global atrophy was seen. The interictal EEG showed isolated spikes left central, the ictal EEG recording showed no specific correlation to myoclonias. In the analysis of back-averaging of the myoclonias no EEG correlation was seen.

The authors discussed the hypothesis that the missing correlation from EMG and EEG signal is caused by the localisation of the hyperexcitable region in the cortex (central sulcus, left perirolandic) with the tangential dipole to the surface EEG and projection to the brainstem.

Findings with imaging

MR imaging in RE

MRI is nonrevealing in primary RE, whereas variable lesions were seen in patients with secondary RE (Koutroumanidis et al., 1998; Mayer, unpublished data, 2001):

- Stroke with left temporoparietal infarction.
- Stroke with left frontal infarction.
- Arachnoidal cyst, left temporal.
- Lesion in left basal ganglia.
- Schizencephaly, left.
- Cavernoma, left frontal.
- Hippocampal sclerosis, right.
- Malformation, left frontal.

Functional imaging in RE

Only patients with secondary RE and localised lesions have been investigated by *interictal* HMPAO-SPECT or PET. In all cases the authors (Koepp et al., 1998; Miyamoto et al., 1995) found hypometabolism in the area of the lesion.

Ictal PET was investigated by Koepp and co-workers (1998). They found a significant reduced binding of 11 C-DPN with opioid receptors in different regions:

- Left parieto-temporo-occipital (Brodmann's area 37).
- Left gyrus temporalis medialis (Brodmann's area 21).
- Parieto-occipital posterior bilateral (Brodmann's area 40).

They did not find any significant opioid release at the Wernicke area.

Ictal HMPAO-SPECT findings showed focal hyperperfusion frontal bilateral and left temporal (Miyamoto et al., 1995).

Juvenile myoclonic epilepsy (JME)

Definition: "JME appears around puberty and is characterized by seizures with bilateral, single or repetitive, arrhythmic, irregular myoclonic jerks, predominantly in the arms. Jerks may cause some patients to fall suddenly. No disturbance of consciousness is noticeable. The disorder may be inherited, and sex distribution is equal. Often there are GTCS and, less often, infrequent absences. The seizures usually occur shortly after awakening and are often precipitated by sleep deprivation. Interictal and ictal EEG have rapid, generalised, often irregular spike-waves and polyspike-waves; there is no close phase correlation between EEG spikes and jerks. Frequently, the patients are photosensitive. Response to appropriate drugs is good." (Commission, 1989).

Seizure triggers are sudden awakening, sleep deprivation, stress and alcohol. Valproic acid (VPA) is the antiepileptic drug (AED) of choice. The prognosis is good, but some authors believe that in 90% of all cases a lifelong AED therapy is required (Calleja et al., 2001). The age at onset is typically between 12 and 18 years. The typical EEG features are generalised spike-waves and polyspike-waves, but also focal epileptic discharges in up to 36% (Lancman et al., 1997). At least one-third of the patients are photosensitive (Wolf & Goosses, 1986).

Panzica and co-workers (2001) investigated the cortical myoclonus in JME with jerk-related back-averaging on ictal epochs. They concluded that the ultimate mechanism responsible for ictal myoclonic jerks in JME is largely similar to that sustaining cortical myoclonus in more severe pathological conditions such as progressive myoclonus epilepsy.

■ Own investigations

Between 1990 and 2001, we investigated six patients with primary RE with an age at onset from 13 to 23 years. In all but one, we found PORM induced by reading and also by speaking. One patient reported a strange, difficult-to-describe feeling in the throat with an inability to read on. This feeling was induced only by reading. PORM in the other five patients showed a tendency to the right side, but even in individual patients the jerks could change lateralisation. GTCS appeared in four of the six patients. Also in four of the six patients, focal (left temporal or frontal) ictal epileptic discharges were observed. VPA was the drug of choice. We saw five seizure-free patients in this group, all of them treated with VPA with a follow-up of one year or more. One patient did not want any medication; she occasionally has PORM but no GTCS. Since the confirmation of the diagnosis, she stops reading when repetitive PORM occur and has thus remained free of GTCS for six years.

In an analysis of all cases with PORM in our centre, we identified 24 patients with PORM between 1994 and 1998, ten with symptomatic focal epilepsies, two with idiopathic generalised epilepsy (IGE) with GM on awakening and twelve with JME. After the diagnosis of PORM in twelve patients with JME, we conducted a questionnaire survey for all our ambulatory patients with the diagnosis JME to search for this and other reflex epileptic traits. The questionnaire was sent to 86 patients, and 65 (75%) responded. Not considering nonspecific precipitating mechanisms, 33 of these patients answered "yes" to questions about specific precipitating stimuli. These patients were investigated by prolonged polygraphic video-EEG recording and were compared with a control group (matched pairs, with different types of epilepsies other than JME).

We performed a standardized interview with all patients, a video-EEG investigation lasting three hours as a minimum, including five minutes hyperventilation, intermittent light stimulation and complex neuropsychological tests. These followed, with modifications, the neuropsychological EEG activation procedure as published by Matsuoka et al. (2000) and comprised the following:

- Reading silently (15 min., standardised text).
- Reading aloud (15 min., standardised text).
- Speaking (about the epilepsy, medical history).
- Mental calculations, e.g. 11 × 11; 125 / 5.
- Written calculation: e.g. 15 × 67 × 23 × 48.
- Writing of standardised texts.
- Spatial constructions, drawing figures, block design test.

Between two tests, there was always a resting time of 15 minutes.

Results of standardised investigations in JME

Questionnaire

The questionnaire, which was sent to all outpatients with JME (see above), provided the following data:

Seven of the 33 positive responses concerned seizure precipitation by intermittent light stimuli. Twenty-one responses referred to "praxis" and comprised stimuli such as writing (8), decision-making (3), computer tasks and video games (6), calculations (6), thinking (8), and playing the piano (1). Seventeen patients reported PORM precipitated by talking (delivering a speech in five), and nine of them by reading. Eleven patients reported about precipitation by both praxis and talking/reading.

Video-EEG investigation

We investigated until now 22 of the 33 patients who had reported on specific seizure precipitation in the questionnaire, and compared them with 20 matched control persons. The mean age of the JME patients was 28.6; the mean age of the control group was 29.2 years. A female predominance was obvious in both groups (10 males *versus* 12 females in the JME group; 8 males *versus* 12 females in the control group). In the control group 15 patients suffered from focal epilepsy, five from generalised epilepsy.

Interictal EEG (*Figure 1*)

We saw a statistically significant difference (Fisher's exact test, two-tailed) in two items: 16 patients in the JME group *versus* four patients in the control group had generalised epileptic discharges, whereas five patients in the JME group *versus* no patient in the control group had focal discharges.

EEG activation (*Figure 2*)

There was a significant difference (Fisher's exact test, one-tailed) between the JME patients and the control group, comparing the precipitation of epileptic discharges during the EEG recording. Nine patients in the JME group, and one in the control

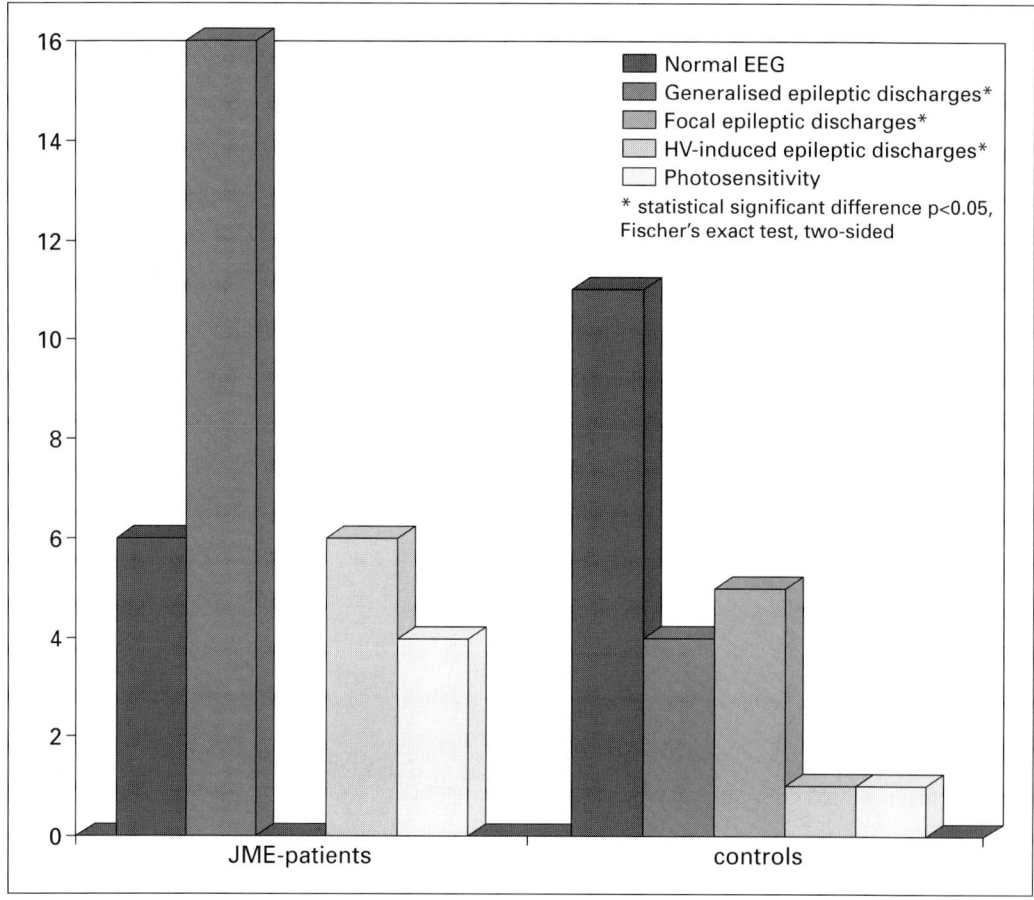

Figure 1. Interictal EEG recording.
JME: juvenile myoclonic epilepsy; HV: hyperventilation.
* Statistical significant difference p < 0.05, Fisher's exact test, two-sided.

group, had epileptic discharges induced by reading or speaking. Six of the patients with JME had praxis-induced epileptic discharges; none of the control group had such discharges.

Precipitation of PORM *(Figure 3)*

In seven of the patients with JME we recorded PORM induced by reading and speaking. Only one patient of the control group had this trait. This difference was also statistically significant (Fisher's exact test, one-tailed). Three of these patients, all with JME, also had praxis-induced seizures. Due to the small number of patients, this difference was not significant (Fisher's exact test, one-tailed).

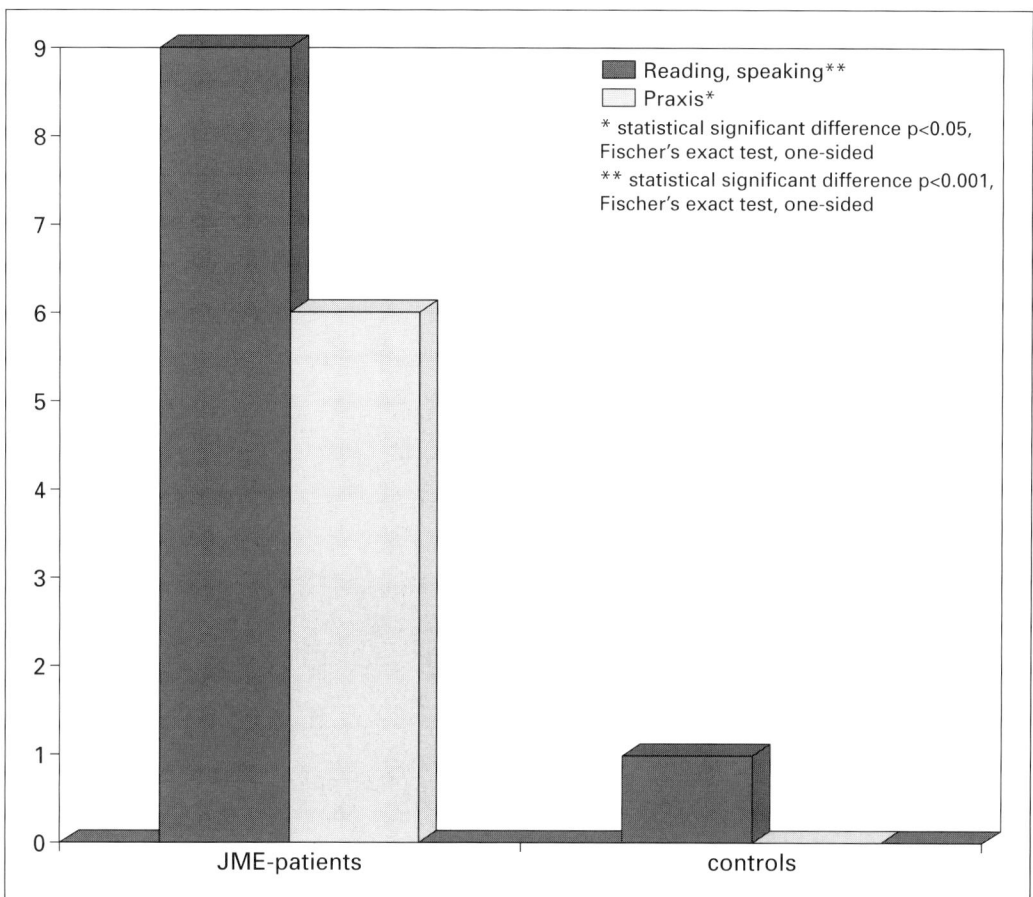

Figure 2. Induced epileptic discharges. (Induction of epileptic discharges by reading/speaking/praxis of more than 200% per time unit in comparison to baseline EEG recording at rest.)
* Statistical significant difference $p < 0.05$, Fisher's exact test, one-sided.
** Statistical significant difference $p < 0.001$, Fisher's exact test, one-sided.

Semiology of PORM

We compared the semiology of PORM in patients with primary RE (n = 6) and those with JME (n = 3). We observed that "PORM plus" only occurred in patients with JME, but this difference was not significant due to the small number of patients. The typical jerks in the perioral muscles did not show differences in both epilepsy syndromes.

Treatment (Figure 4)

Therapy was easy in patients with primary RE. All responded very well to VPA; only one patient decided not to take any medication. She has been seizure-free for more than five years, having learned to interrupt reading when frequent PORM occur.

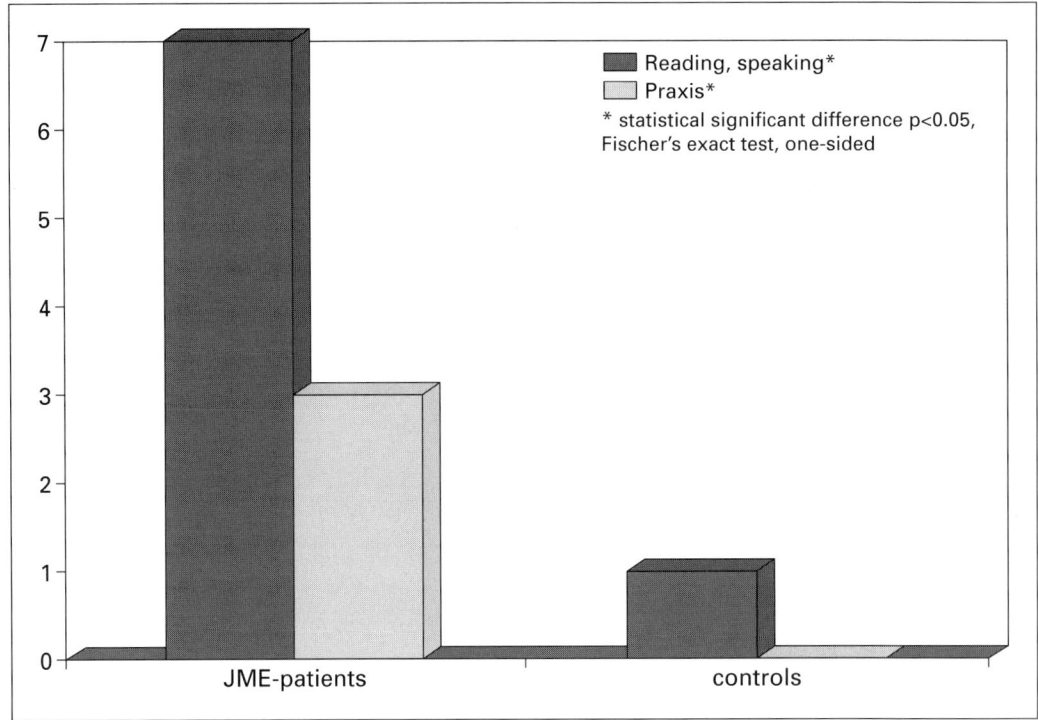

Figure 3. Induced epileptic seizures.
* Statistical significant difference p < 0.05, Fisher's exact test, one-sided.

Three of the patients with JME and PORM were not seizure-free with VPA; only one did not respond at all, the other 18 were seizure-free with VPA. This contrasts with "secondary RE", i.e. a somewhat heterogeneous group of 10 patients suffering from focal symptomatic epilepsies with PORM. One patient became seizure-free with carbamazepine (CBZ); another one experienced a seizure reduction of more than 50% with CBZ. The others were difficult to treat, and PORM even sometimes persisted when other seizures responded to treatment.

■ Discussion

In the database Medline we found 250 published papers between 1979 and 2001 dealing with JME. Only a few papers dealt with special investigations on reflex epileptic traits (Inoue et al., 1994, 2000; Matsuoka et al., 2000). We found 149 papers about RE, but only one paper was dealing with PORM in patients with JME (Radhakrishan et al., 1995).

These authors described 18 patients with RE, four of whom also had a diagnosis of JME. Three of them were female. The age at onset was from 14 to 17 years; one patient was 46 years old at the beginning of RE. The triggers of seizures in all patients were reading, in three patients also calculations. Listening to conservation, playing chess or speaking were triggers in individual cases. The interictal and ictal EEG

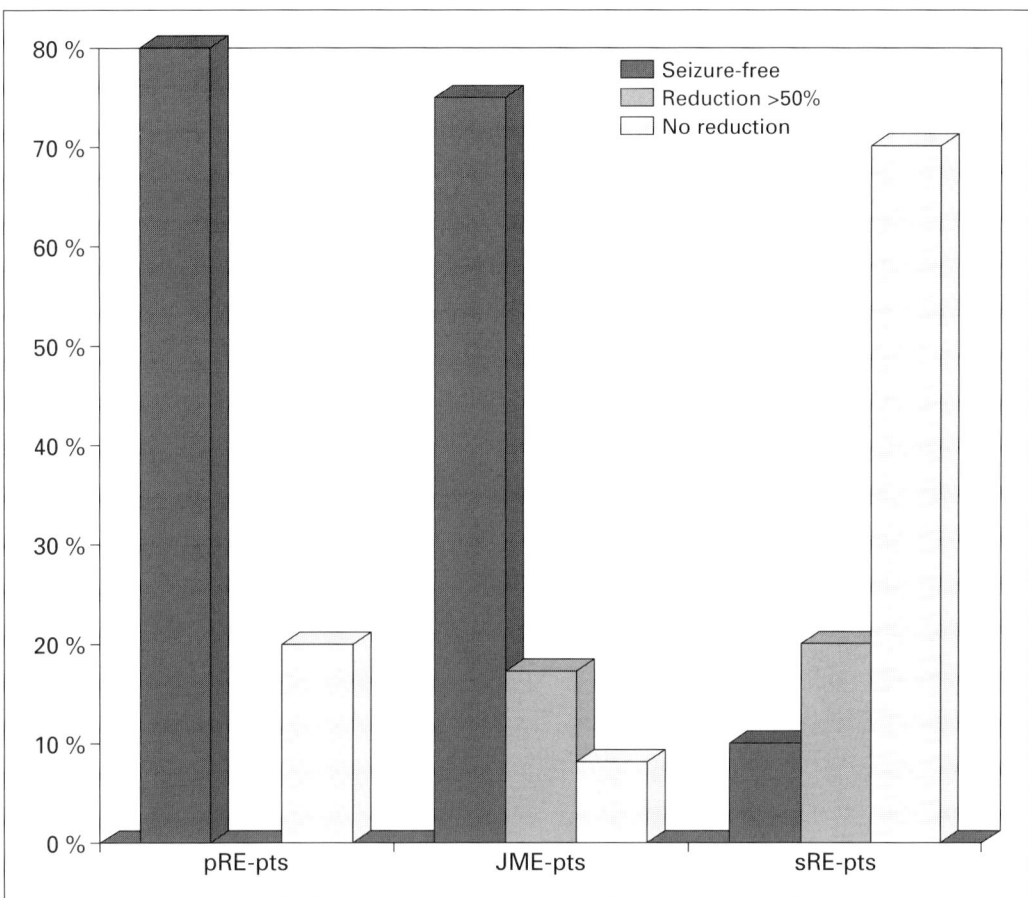

Figure 4. Treatment of patients with PRM (Perioral Reflex Myoclonia).
pRE: primary reading epilepsy; JME: juvenile myoclonic epilepsy; sRE: secondary reading epilepsy.

showed generalised epileptic discharges in all patients; none of the patients was photosensitive. Two of them responded to VPA, partial control was seen in two patients treated with phenytoin and primidone.

Matsuoka et al. (2000) investigated 480 patients with different kinds of epileptic syndromes with a specially designed neuropsychological EEG activation program. This program consisted of different tasks including reading and speaking (both very brief), arithmetic, writing, drawing and the block design test. In 133 patients an inhibitory effect of activation was seen in the EEG. In 38 patients, activation induced epileptic discharges, most of them in response to mental or written calculation (n = 21), writing of special standardized sentences (n = 26) or spatial constructions (n = 24). Only in two of the 38 patients was reading a specific trigger; none of them had speaking-induced seizures.

Concerning the relation of these findings to epilepsy syndromes, Matsuoka and co-workers found that all but two of the patients who responded to activation had idiopathic generalised syndromes. Most of them (n = 22) had JME, only two patients had temporal lobe seizures. Considering the semiology of precipitated seizures they found that in most cases (n = 32) these were myoclonic seizures in both arms; 23 had GTCS, 19 had absence seizures, two patients had secondarily GTCS, and two had partial seizures. PORM were not seen in any of the patients, probably because the patients read and talked too little. Another reason for the missing PORM in this work could be that patients and investigators were not aware of the short PORM which often have no EEG correlate but a short EMG artefact.

Inoue and co-workers (2000) investigated patients with JME with a special test battery to search for praxis-induced seizures (PIS). Such seizures are triggered by a complex interaction of thinking with a manual task. Several of their patients had seizures while doing calculations with the traditional Japanese abacus, the "soroban". This activity is a perfect example of praxis in the sense of a differentiated manual task guided by cognition, and the usually rapid performance enhances the stimulus. Most of the investigated 213 patients were photosensitive (n = 47). In 20 patients typing or writing was provocative. In 16 patients playing cards or chess precipitated myoclonic jerks in the active arm. Mental or written calculation was provocative in 15 patients, complicated finger manipulation in eleven. Only a few patients responded to playing video games (n = 6) or playing musical instruments (n = 4). PORM were reported in none of the patients.

All these patients have in common that some local motor activity on which the patients' attention is focused provokes local myoclonic phenomena or, as Bickford put it in his first description of RE, that "proprioceptive bombardment" that results in "reflex firing through the same motor segment" (Bickford et al., 1956). It is surprising that these minimal partial motor seizures happen both in a condition which is considered a "generalised" epilepsy syndrome (JME) and a localisation-related epilepsy syndrome (RE). Furthermore, the reflex-like phenomena we observed here look substantially different from the typical bilateral brachial jerks of JME. The reflex epileptic seizure symptoms remain restricted to rather circumscribed areas. It is an intriguing question how rather direct, local reflex-like sensorimotor interactions fit into a "generalised" syndrome.

Perhaps this is the right place to remember that it is a mere convention to call the bilateral motor manifestations in JME "generalised" just because the concomitant EEG shows widespread polyspike-waves. The seizure semiology, however, is restricted to a rather circumscribed, albeit bilateral area.

At the Bethel-Cleveland Symposium of 1993 (Wolf, 1994), many of the contributions and discussions dealt with the relation of the widespread bilateral discharges, which by convention are today called "generalised", to the (bilateral or unilateral) regional expression of clinical symptoms. This discussion needs perhaps to be pursued. One of the open questions in this respect is, in photosensitive JME patients, by what intermediaries the occipital cortical input of intermittent lights produces myoclonic jerks of the extremities. Still, these are bilateral and roughly symmetric.

These observations seem to indicate that the distinction between focal and generalised epileptic phenomena may to some extent be artificial. The closer we look at the prototype of an idiopathic generalised epilepsy syndrome, JME, the more we have to realise, so it seems, that it is indeed a syndrome which challenges our syndromic concepts.

The next steps to a better understanding of the pathophysiology of PORM will be functional imaging (fMRI) in patients with JME and RE during reading provocation to look for the brain activity in comparison to normal controls (Price *et al.*, 1994).

Conclusion

PORM are obvious but often unrecognised focal seizures in different epileptic syndromes, and the leading seizure type in reading epilepsy. They are frequent in JME compared with other epilepsy syndromes. Photosensitivity and PORM are usually not present in some patients. PORM remain often undiagnosed because the patients are not aware that they are epileptic, and fail to report them. Their semiology is not fundamentally different in various epileptic syndromes. However, it seems that the "PORM plus" perhaps do not occur in RE. PORM are symptoms in different epileptic syndromes, where they indicate locally much restricted epileptic activity. These observations seem to indicate that the distinction between focal and generalised epileptic phenomena may be less clear than is traditionally believed. VPA seems to be the AED of choice in most cases of both primary RE and of PORM in JME. Their response to AEDs in other epilepsy syndromes remains to be better investigated.

References

1. Atassi M. Primäre Lese-Epilepsie. Eine Kasuistik. *Z. EEG-EMG* 1981; 12: 128-31.
2. Bartolomei F, Farnarier G, Elias Z, Bronsard G, Soulayrol S, Bonnet A, Chave B, Gastaut JL. Facial reflex myoclonus induced by language: a neuropsychological and neurophysiological study. *Neurophysiol Clin* 1999; 29: 263-70.
3. Baxter DW, Bailey AA. Primary reading epilepsy. *Neurology* 1961; 11: 445-9.
4. Bennett DR, Mavor H, Jarcho LW. Language-inducted epilepsy: report of a case. *Electroencephalogr Clin Neurophysiol* 1971; 30: 159.
5. Berendes K, Mattes W, Dörstelmann D. Medikamentöse Behandlung der Leseepilepsie. *Nervenarzt* 1983; 54: 435-6.
6. Bickford RG. Discussion. *Trans Am Neurol Ass* 1973; 98: 187-8.
7. Bickford RG, Whelan JL, Klass DW, Corbin KB. Reading epilepsy: clinical and electroencephalographic studies of a new syndrome. *Trans Am Neurol Ass* 1956; 81: 100-2.
8. Bingel A. Reading epilepsy. *Neurology* 1957; 7: 752-6.
9. Borusiak P, Mayer Th. West Syndrom und Leseepilepsie: Eine Kasuistik zu idiopathischen fokalen Epilepsien. In: Stephani U, ed. *Aktuelle Neuropädiatrie 2000.* Novartis Pharma Verlag, Nürnberg, 2001; 105-8.
10. Brooks JE, Jirauch PM. Primary reading epilepsy. A misnomer. *Arch Neurol* 1971; 25: 97-104.
11. Calleja S, Salas-Puig J, Ribacoba R, Lahoz CH. Evolution of juvenile myoclonic epilepsy treated from the outset with sodium valproate. *Seizure* 2001; 10 (6): 424-7.

12. Canevini MP, Vignoli A, Sgro V, Zambrelli E, Piazini A, Colombo N, Canger R. Symptomatic epilepsy with facial myoclonus triggered by language. *Epil Dis* 2001; 3/3: 143-6.
13. Christie S, Guberman A, Tansley BW, Couture M. Primary reading epilepsy: investigation of critical seizure-provoking stimuli. *Epilepsia* 1988; 26: 288-93.
14. Chritchley M, Cobb W, Sears TA. On reading epilepsy. *Epilepsia* 1959; 1: 403-17.
15. Cirignotta F, Zucconi M, Mondini S, Lugaresi E. Writing epilepsy. *Clin Electroencephalogr* 1986; 17: 21-3.
16. Cohn R, Allison ME, De Bolt WL. Reading epilepsy. Electroencephalogr. *Clin Neurophysiol* 1961; 13: 315.
17. Commission on Classification and Terminology of the International League against Epilepsy Proposal for revised classification of epilepsies and epileptic syndromes. *Epilepsia* 1989; 30: 389-99.
18. Daly RF, Forster FM. Inheritance of reading epilepsy. *Neurology* 1975; 25: 1051-4.
19. Forster FM, Daly RF. Reading epilepsy in identical twins. *Trans Am Neurol Ass* 1973; 98: 186-8.
20. Forstner G, Ferguson R, Jones DP. Reading epilepsy. *Can Med Assoc J* 1961; 85: 608-9.
21. Gastaut H, Tassinari C. Triggering mechanisms in epilepsy. The electroclinical point of view. *Epilepsia* 1966; 7: 85-138.
22. Geschwind N, Sherwin I. Language-induced epilepsy. *Arch Neurol* 1967; 16: 25-31.
23. Gilligan BS. Primary reading epilepsy. *Med J Austral* 1969; 56: 1025-8.
24. Hall JH, Marshall PC. Reply from the authors. *Neurology* 1983; 32: 117-8.
25. Hall JH, Marshall PC. Clonazepam therapy in reading epilepsy. *Arch Neurol* 1980; 16: 25-31.
26. Hallett M, Chadwick D, Marsden CD. Cortical reflex myoclonus. *Neurology* 1979; 8: 1107-25.
27. Hallett M. Myoclonus: relation to epilepsy. *Epilepsia* 1985; 26 (suppl. 1): S67-77.
28. Hiranuma H, Shiraiwa N. A case report of reading epilepsy. *Clin Electroencephalogr* 1978; 20: 565.
29. Hosokawa K, Nishioka H, Yamamoto S. One case of "reading epilepsy". *Psychiatry* 1965; 7: 71-6.
30. Inoue Y, Seino M, Kubota H, Yamakaku K, Tanaka M, Yagi K. Epilepsy with praxis-induced seizures. In: Wolf P, ed. *Epileptic Seizures and Syndromes*. London: John Libbey, 1994; 81-91.
31. Jones EA, Aoki C. The processing of Japanese Kana and Kanji characters. In: de Kerckhove D, Lumsden Ch J, eds. *The alphabet and in the brain*. Berlin, Heidelberg: Springer, 1988; 301-20.
32. Kartsounis LD. Comprehension as the effective trigger in a case of primary reading epilepsy. *J Neurol Neurosurg Psychiatr* 1988; 51: 128-30.
33. Koepp MJ, Hansen ML, Pressler R, Brooks DJ, Brandl U, Guldin B, Duncan JS, Ried S. Comparison of EEG, MRI and PET in reading epilepsy: a case report. *Epil Res* 1998; 29: 251-7.
34. Koepp MJ, Richardson MP, Brooks DJ, Friston KJ, Duncan JS. [11 C]-Diprenorphine activation study in patients with reading epilepsy. *Epilepsia* 1995; 36 (suppl. 3): 138.
35. Koutroumanidis M, Koepp MJ, Richardson MP, Camfield C, Agathonikou A, Ried S, Papadimitriou A, Plant GT, Duncan JS, Panayiatopoulos CP. The variants of reading epilepsy. *Brain* 1998; 121: 1409-27.
36. Krause KH. Primäre Leseepilepsie. Ein kasuistischer Beitrag. *Nervenarzt* 1977; 48: 285-8.
37. Lancman ME, Asconape JJ, Penry JK. Clinical and EEG asymmetries in juvenile myoclonic epilepsy. *Epilepsia* 1997; 38 (2): 258.
38. Lasater GM. Reading epilepsy. *Arch Neurol* 1962; 6: 492-5.
39. Lee SJ, Sutherling WW, Persing JA, Butler AB. Language-induced seizure. A case of cortical origin. *Arch Neurol* 1980; 37: 433-6.
40. Login JS, Kolakovich TM. Successful treatment of primary reading epilepsy with clonazepam. *Ann Neurol* 1978; 4: 155-6.
41. Matricardi M, Brinciotti M, Paciello F. Reading epilepsy with absences, television-induced seizures, and pattern sensitivity. *Epilepsy Res* 1991; 9: 145-7.

42. Matsuoka H, Takahashi T, Sasaki M, Matsumoto K, Yoshida S, Numachi Y, Saito H, Ueno T, Sato M. Neuropsychological EEG activation in patients with epilepsy. *Brain* 2000; 123: 318-30.
43. Matthews WB, Wright FK. Hereditary primary reading epilepsy. *Neurology* 1967; 17: 919-21.
44. Mayer T, Wolf P. Reading epilepsy: Related to Juvenile Myoclonic epilepsy? *Epilepsia* 1997; 38 (suppl. 3): 18-9.
45. Mayer T, Wolf P. Reading epilepsy: clinical and genetic background. In: Berkovic S, Genton P, Marescaux C, Picard F, eds. *Genetics of Focal Epilepsies: Clinical Aspects and Molecular Biology*. London: John Libbey, 1999; 159-67.
46. Mayer T, Wolf P. Perioral Reflex-Myoclonia: A frequent seizure-type. Analysis of 28 patients with reading-induced seizures. *Epilepsia* 1999; 40 (suppl. 2): 21-2.
47. Mayer T, Schroeder F, Wolf P. Reflex epileptic traits in juvenile myoclonic epilepsy. *Epilepsia* 2001; 42 (suppl. 2): 176-7.
48. Mayersdorf A, Marshall C. Pattern activation in reading epilepsy. A case of report. *Epilepsia* 1970; 11: 423-6.
49. Mesri JC, Pagano MA. Reading epilepsy. *Epilepsia* 1987; 28: 301-4.
50. Meyer JG, Wolf P. Über primäre Leseepilepsie. Mit einem kasuistischen Beitrag. *Nervenarzt* 1973; 44: 155-60.
51. Miyamoto A, Takahashi S, Tokumitsu A, Oki J. Ictal HMPAO-Single Photon Emission Computed Tomography Findings in Reading Epilepsy in a Japanese Boy. *Epilepsia* 1995; 36: 1161-3.
52. Murphy MJ, Yamada T. Clonazepam therapy in reading epilepsy. *Neurology* 1981; 31: 233.
53. Newmann PK, Longly BP. Reading epilepsy. *Arch Neurol* 1984; 41: 13-4.
54. Norbury FB, Loeffler JD. Primary reading epilepsy. *JAMA* 1963; 194: 661-2.
55. Obeso JA, Rothwell JC, Marden CD. The spectrum of cortical myoclonus. From focal reflex jerks to spontaneous motor epilepsy. *Brain* 1985; 108 (Part 1): 193-224.
56. Panzica F, Rubboli G, Franceschetti S, Avanzini G, Meletti S, Pozzi A, Tassinari CA. Cortical myoclonus in Janz Syndrome. *Clin Neurophysiol* 2001; 112: 1803-9.
57. Price CJ, Wise RJS, Watson JDG, Patterson K, Howard D, Frackowiak RSJ. Brain activity during reading. *Brain* 1994; 117: 1255-69.
58. Radhakrishan K, Silbert PL, Klass DW. Reading epilepsy. An appraisal of 20 patients diagnosed at the Mayo Clinic, Rochester, Minnesota, between 1949 and 1989, and delineation of the epileptic syndrome. *Brain* 1995; 118: 75-89.
59. Ramani V. Reading Epilepsy. In: Zifkin BJ, Andermann F, Beaumanoir A, Rowan AJ, eds. *Reflex Epilepsies and Reflex Seizures. Advances in Neurology* 1998; vol. 75: 241-62.
60. Ramani V. Primary reading epilepsy. *Arch Neurol* 1983; 40: 39-41.
61. Ried S, Behl I, Schmidt D. Leseepilepsie: eine Variante des Impulsiv-Petit mal? In: Scheffner D, ed. *Epilepsie 90*. Reinbeck: Einhorn-Presse, 1991; 168-73.
62. Ritaccio AL, Hickling EJ, Ramani V. The Role of Dominant Premotor Cortex and Grapheme to Phoneme Transformation in Reading Epilepsy. *Archives of Neurology* 1992; 49: 933-9.
63. Rowan AJ, Heathfield KGW, Scott DF. Is reading epilepsy inherited? *J Neurol Neurosurg Psychiatry* 1970; 33: 476-8.
64. Saenz-Lope E, Herranz-Tanarro FJ, Masdeu JC. Primary reading epilepsy. *Epilepsia* 1985; 26: 649-56.
65. Schomer DL, Pegna A, Matton B, Seeck M, Bidaut L, Slossmann D, Roth S, Landis T. Ictal agraphia: A patient study. *Neurology* 1998; 50: 542-5.
66. Stella L, Fels A, Pillo G, Fragassi N, Buscanio GA, Striano S. Primary reading epilepsy. Clinical and EEG study of a case and characteristics of the effective stimulus. *Acta Neurol Napoli* 1983; 5: 426-31.
67. Taylor MM. The bilateral cooperative model of reading. In: De Kerckhove D, Lumsden Ch J, eds. *The alphabet and in the brain*. Berlin, Heidelberg: Springer, 1988; 322-61.

68. Vanderzant Ch, Fitz R, Holmes G, Greenberg HS, Sackellares J Ch. Treatment of primary reading epilepsy with Valproic Acid. *Arch Neurol* 1982; 39: 452-3.
69. Watson P. Clonazepam therapy in reading epilepsy. *Neurology* 1983; 32: 117.
70. Wolf P. Reading epilepsy. In: Wolf P, ed. *Epileptic Seizures and Syndromes*. London: John Libbey, 1994; 67-74.
71. Wolf P, Goosses R. Relation of photosensitivity to epileptic syndromes. *J Neurol Neurosurg Psychiatry* 1986; **49**: 1386-91.
72. Wolf P. Reading epilepsy: evidence for a cognitive factor in seizure precipitation. In: Meinradi H, Rowan AJ, eds. *Advances in epileptology*. Amsterdam, Lisse: Swets Zeitlinger, 1978; 85-90.
73. Wolf P, Goosses R. Relation of photosensitivity to epileptic syndromes. *J Neurol Neurosurg Psychiat* 1986; 49: 1386-91.
74. Wolf P. Reflex epilepsies and syndrome classification. An argument for considering primary reading epilepsy as an idiopathic localization-related epilepsy. In: Beaumanoir A, Gastaut H, Naquet R, eds. *Reflex seizures and reflex epilepsies*. Genève: Médecine et Hygiène, 1989; 283-6.
75. Wolf P. Reading epilepsy. In: Roger J, Bureau M, Dravet Ch, Dreyfuss FE, Perret A, Wolf P, eds. *Epileptic syndromes in infancy, childhood and adolescence* (2nd edition). 1992; 281-98.
76. Wolf P, ed. *Epileptic seizures and Syndromes*. London: John Libbey, 1994.
77. Wolf P, Mayer T, Reker M. Reading epilepsy: Report of five new cases and further considerations on the pathophysiology. *Seizure* 1998; 7: 271-9.
78. Wolf P, Mayer T. Juvenile Myoclonic Epilepsy: A Syndrome Challenging Syndromic Concepts. In: Schmitz B, Sander T, eds. *Juvenile Myoclonic Epilepsy: the Janz Syndrome*. Whrightson Biomedical Publishing Ltd. Petersfield, UK, Philadelphia, USA, 2000; 33-40.
79. Yalçin AD, Forta H. Primary reading epilepsy. *Seizure* 1998; 7: 325-7.

▪ Ictal SPECT investigation

Background

Ictal radioisotope studies are difficult to perform and limited by the low temporal resolution in SPECT and PET. Patients with reading epilepsy, however, may reliably provoke seizures in the scanner and thus, radioisotope studies may provide insights into the cerebral pathophysiology and neurochemistry of such activity.

Rationale. To clarify the ictal region of brain involvement in a 14-year-old Japanese boy with reading epilepsy (Miyamato *et al.*, 1995).

Methods

Ictal SPECT with [99mTc] hexamethylpropylene amine oxime (HMPAO) was performed in a 14-year-old Japanese boy. Five minutes after jaw jerking began, HMPAO was administered intravenously and the boy continued reading for two more minutes. HMPAO SPECT at rest was also performed. A healthy 25-year-old woman was studied twice, with reading and at rest, for comparison.

Results and Discussion

Interictal HMPAO SPECT did not show significant asymmetries. Ictal SPECT revealed hyperperfusion in both frontal lobes, more notable in the left, and also within the left temporal lobe. Meaningful interpretation of the findings was difficult as the healthy control also showed left frontotemporal hyperperfusion, albeit to a lesser degree and extent. The ictal EEG in this patient was characterised by bilateral spike-wave complexes with a left frontotemporal predominance and in a similar distribution to the ictal SPECT findings.

▪ Ictal PET investigation

Background

FMRI and BOLD contrast or HMPAO-SPECT activation studies measure changes in regional cerebral blood flow (rCBF) which only reflect local synaptic activity. Neurotransmitters are responsible for mediating neuronal activity. Endogenous neurotransmitter release is a pivotal event in neuroregulation, but has been very difficult to study noninvasively *in vivo* in man. To date, PET studies of neurotransmitter release in humans have concentrated on pharmacological manipulations and measured changes in receptor availability to radioligands. The detection of endogenous neurotransmitter release using PET relies on the kinetic behaviour of a high affinity PET tracer being disturbed by endogenous neurotransmitters with much lower affinities given significant changes in occupancy and concentrations of available binding sites.

Rationale. To study dynamic neurotransmitter changes in specific brain areas in relation to focal epileptic seizures (Koepp *et al.*, 1998a).

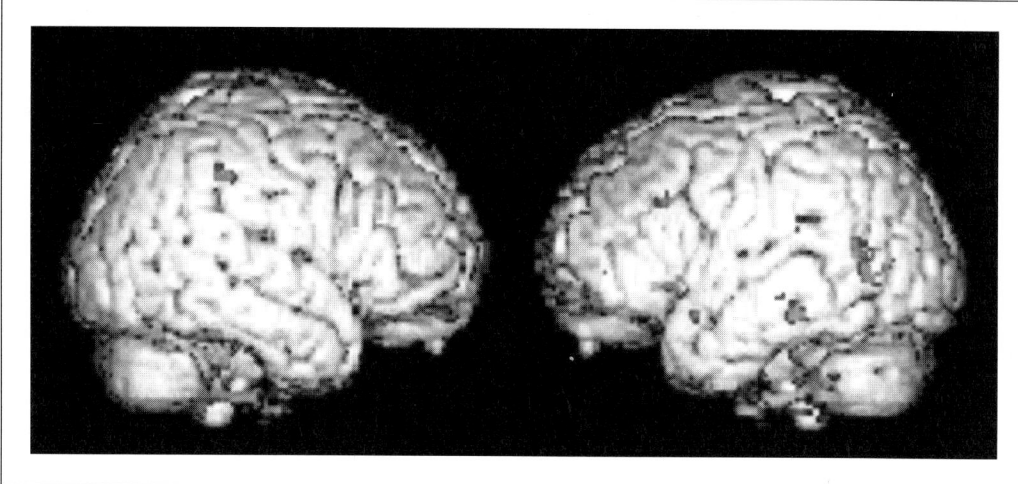

Figure 3. Statistical parametric map showing areas of reduced DPN binding (p < 0.05 corrected) during reading-induced seizures.

Methods

Five patients with reading epilepsy and six healthy controls were studied twice with a pair of dynamic 90-minute high-resolution ^{11}C-diprenorphine (DPN) PET scans. During the first scan 30 minutes post-injection, subjects were asked to read aloud from a screen. Four of the five patients thus experienced focal seizures consisting of short jaw jerks and/or dysphasia. During the second scan subjects were asked to study a list of meaningless symbols for the same period of time without provoking any seizure activity. Using spectral analysis (Cunningham & Jones, 1993), parametric images of cerebral DPN binding were calculated for both scans. For all five patients and six controls the differences between DPN binding during reading/seizures *versus* looking at symbols/rest were compared on a voxel-by-voxel basis using SPM. If reading DPN binding of the reading scan was lower than resting DPN binding, displacement of the radioactive DPN by an endogenous release of an opioid-like substance would be implied.

Results and discussion

No significant differences were found when comparing rest scans and reading scans in both controls and patients. Furthermore, there was no difference in resting opioid binding between patients and controls. Significant reductions in patient DPN binding (p < 0.001 corrected) were observed when comparing the interaction of rest minus activation between patient and control groups *(Figure 3)*. The most significant areas of reduced DPN binding were within the left parieto-temporo-occipital cortex (BA 37). Other areas displaying reduced DPN binding at lower significance (p < 0.001 uncorrected) included the left middle temporal gyrus (BA 21) and the posterior parieto-occipital junction (BA 40).

These results suggest endogenous opioids to be released in a specific neuronal network involved in reading, visual processing and recognition of words. The left posterior temporal and the left inferior parietal cortex have recently both been shown to be associated with word processing. Both, the "ventral and dorsal streams" appear to be involved in the physiological processing of reading. The "dorsal stream" of projections from striate cortex to posterior parietal regions is likely to be involved in encoding the spatial coordinates of words and sentences. Projections along the "ventral stream" to the left inferotemporal cortex are associated with complex semantic judgement and sentence comprehension.

Conclusions

Functional neuroimaging has had until now a limited impact on our understanding of the pathophysiological and neurochemical abnormalities underlying reading epilepsy with only a few existing reports in the literature (Miyamato et al., 1995; Koepp et al., 1998a; Archer et al., 2001). We previously reported direct *in vivo* PET evidence for the dynamic multifocal release of endogenous opioids during and following reading-induced partial seizures in areas known to be involved in reading, visual processing and word recognition (Koepp et al., 1998a). The most significant area of reduced DPN binding during reading-induced seizures are in close proximity to areas found to be hypoactive in the same patients on fMRI during normal reading. These cortical and subcortical areas may both represent hyperexcitable cortex, and constitute part of the normal reading network. Recruitment of a "critical mass" of such an area with synchronisation and subsequent spreading of excitation in response to the epileptogenic stimulus could precipitate epileptiform EEG activity or a clinical seizure. Increasing the complexity of epileptogenic stimuli may facilitate such a recruitment (Koepp et al., 1998b). This recruitment may involve the participation and interaction of several cortical and subcortical structures activated by reading, and need not be confined to physically contiguous brain sites or established neuronal links. It may rely on both existing and reorganised functional links between brain regions. The reported observations are consistent with this concept of variable hyperexcitability at multiple cortical and subcortical levels allowing for any asymmetric or symmetric generalised ictal EEG discharge, regional and focal discharges. This theory can also explain the heterogeneity of clinical phenomena encountered and efficacy of various linguistic stimuli as seizure triggers (Koutroumanidis et al., 1998). Functional imaging studies with larger cohorts are clearly required to elucidate this further.

Summary

The neuroanatomical and biochemical basis of reading epilepsy is largely unknown and structural neuroimaging is usually normal. Functional neuroimaging, using functional magnetic resonance imaging (fMRI), single photon emission computed tomography (SPECT) and positron emission tomography (PET), allows for localising changes in cerebral blood flow, metabolism and neurotransmitter levels that accompany changes in neural activity. Ictal investigations are difficult to perform due to the paroxysmal nature of the epilepsies. Reflex epilepsies, such as reading epilepsy, are thus an ideal model to study functional changes that occur at or around the time of seizures. In addition, functional imaging in reflex epilepsies may help identify neuronal and cognitive reorganisation. This should increase our understanding of both the pathophysiology and spatial distribution of networks underlying epileptiform activity, and the reciprocal relationship between epileptic activity and cognition. We recently found evidence for the release of endogenous opioids during and following reading-induced partial seizures in areas of the brain involved in normal reading (Koepp et al., 1998). This led to the hypothesis that there are networks of cortical areas concurrently subserving both cognitive functions and epileptic activity.

References

1. Allen PJ, Josephs O, Turner R. A Method for Removing Imaging Artifact from Continuous in reading epilepsy EEG Recorded during Functional MRI. *NeuroImage* 2000; 12: 230-9.
2. Archer JS, Briellmann RS, Syngeniottis A, Abbott DF, Jackson GD. Spike-triggered fMRI in reading epilepsy: involvement of left frontal cortex working memory area. *Neurology* 2003; 60: 415-21.
3. Cunningham VJ, Jones T. Spectral analysis of dynamic PET data. *J Cereb Blood Flow Metab* 1993; 13: 15-23.
4. Fletcher PC, McKenna PJ, Frith CD, Grasby PM, Friston KJ, Dolan RJ. Brain activations in schizophrenia during a graded memory task studied with functional neuroimaging. *Arch Gen Psychiatry* 1998; 55: 1001-8.
5. Koepp MJ, Richardson MP, Brooks DJ, Duncan JS. Focal cortical release of endogenous opioids during reading-induced seizures. *Lancet* 1998a; 352: 952-5.
6. Koepp MJ, Hansen ML, Pressler RM, Brooks DJ, Brandl U, Duncan JS, Ried S. Comparison of EEG, MRI and PET in Reading Epilepsy: a case report. *Epilepsy Research* 1998b; 29: 247-53.
7. Koutroumanidis M, Koepp MJ, Richardson MP, et al. The variants of reading epilepsy. A clinical and video-EEG study of 17 patients with reading-induced seizures. *Brain* 1998; 121: 1409-27.
8. Krakow K, Woermann FG, Symms MR, Allen PJ, Lemieux L, Barker GJ, Duncan JS, Fish DR. EEG-triggered functional MRI of interictal epileptiform activity in patients with focal epilepsy. *Brain* 1999; 122: 1679-88.
9. Miyamato A, Takahashi S, Tokumitsu A, Oki J. Ictal HMPAO-Single Photon Emission Computed Tomography Findings in Reading Epilepsy in a Japanese Boy. *Epilepsia* 1995; 36: 1161-3.
10. Price CJ, Friston KJ. Scanning patients with tasks they can perform. *Human Brain Mapping* 1999; 8: 102-8.
11. Salek-Haddadi A, Hamandi K, Woermann FG, Mayer T, Wolf P, Koepp MJ. Functional MRI in reading epilepsy. *Epilepsia* 2004; 45 (suppl. 3): 64.

Musicogenic seizures and findings on the anatomy of musical perception

H.G. Wieser

Abteilung für Epileptologie & Elektroenzephalographie, Neurologische Klinik, Universitätsspital, Zürich

Introduction

Many stimuli that either induce or precipitate seizures have been delineated and well documented. The mechanisms how they trigger seizures, remain, however, an intriguing and perplexing problem.

What precipitates a seizure at a particular time in the individual epileptic patient? Aird (1983) listed over 40 known epileptogenic mechanisms with some varying from hour to hour depending on the daily activities of the patients. Alterations of level of consciousness, drowsiness and sleep, sleep deprivation, tension states ("stress"), disturbances of water and acid-base balances, sensory stimulation, and drugs and their withdrawal are the principal factors involved. Aird, who studied such seizure-inducing factors prospectively in 500 drug-resistant patients, came to the conclusion that in 17% of his patients such factors were important, insofar as their regulation played a significant role in the stabilisation and improvement of the underlying epileptic condition. But, epileptic seizures that are consistently elicited by a specific stimulus have a prevalence of 4%-7% amongst patients with epilepsies, *i.e.* pure reflex epilepsies are rare (Symonds, 1959).

It is obvious that the importance of the reflex epilepsies is based not so much on their incidence, but on the possibilities to study basic mechanisms of epilepsy, including therapeutic strategies, aimed at inhibiting the focal discharging cortex or the spread of the abnormal discharges along various pathways.

Reflex epilepsies: elementary (simple) versus elaborate (complex) forms

Complex reflex epilepsies are characterized by seizures triggered by relatively elaborate stimuli whose specific pattern is the determining factor in seizure evocation. Integration/alteration of higher cortical functions is important, as is anticipation of the stimulus. Latency from stimulus onset to the clinical or EEG event is typically longer than in simple reflex epilepsies.

Some shared characteristics of the complex reflex epilepsies suggest that recruitment of a "critical mass" of epileptogenic cortex in response to the epileptogenic stimulus can result in epileptiform activity or a clinical seizure. This recruitment may be relatively direct in some cases, but in others the participation and interaction of several cortical areas or of cortex and subcortical structures activated by the external trigger is crucial. Confusion is possible among types of reflex seizures because of the complexity of the triggers.

Complex audiogenic triggers play the decisive role in so-called "musicogenic epilepsy". Reports of patients with seizures habitually precipitated by the voices of radio speakers (Forster et al., 1969) or television performers (Ramani, 1991) remained isolated. In "reading epilepsy" and "language-induced epilepsy" audiogenic triggers may play a role in certain cases. Also in "TV", "Pokemon", and "video game" epilepsies audiogenic triggers might be involved, but visual stimuli are thought to play the crucial role.

■ Musicogenic epilepsy

This type of epilepsy is a rare disorder in which seizures are induced by hearing certain sounds, typically music (Critchley, 1937). Non-musical sounds, such as whirring machinery, can also be effective triggers. An affective component of the stimulus is evident in some patients. In a considerable proportion of the reported cases, seizure precipitation was mediated through a strong emotional factor.

In the majority of patients with "musicogenic epilepsy" the seizures are of simple or complex partial type, with interictal and ictal epileptiform activity recorded from either temporal region (Scott, 1977). We presented arguments that mesiobasal limbic structures play an important role (Wieser & Mazzola, 1986; Wieser et al., 1997; Wieser & Walter, 1997), and that the right temporal lobe is more often involved.

There is often a latency of several minutes during which the patient must be continually exposed to the stimulus for the seizure to occur, and autonomic symptoms and signs may be noted before overt ictal behaviour begins. Patients with musicogenic attacks may also have seizures without audiogenic triggers, *i.e.* so-called "spontaneous" ones.

Reviewing 76 described patients with "musicogenic epilepsy" and adding seven of our own observations, we found the following characteristics in these 83 patients (Tables I-IV): Only 14 patients had exclusively musically triggered fits. Forty-eight patients (out of 62 in whom this information was given) had both musically precipitated seizures and seizures without musical precipitation. In this group of 48 patients

Table I. Review Musicogenic Epilepsy (n 83; 76 patients from literature; 7 own observations): General Characteristics

Information available in n patients			
Sex (n 79)	Males 36	Females 43	
Age at first seizure (n 59)	27.7 ± 12.5 years		
Age at first musically precipitated seizure (n 32)	28.1 ± 9.8 years		
Age at first seizure in patients with *exclusively* musically precipitated seizures (n 14)	32.1 ± 9.3 years		
Coexistence with non-musically precipitated seizures (n 83)	Yes: 48	No: 14	Not stated or uncertain: 21
In patients with spontaneous *and* musically precipitated seizures (n 48) musically precipitated seizures occurred	*Before* spontaneous seizures: 4	*At the same time*: 12	*Later* than spontaneous seizures: 22

Table II. Review Musicogenic Epilepsy (n 83; 76 patients from literature; 7 own observations): Type of Stimulus Precipitating the Seizures

	N 83	Patients with *exclusively* musically triggered seizures (n 14)
Music only	65	12
Classic music	5	1
Predominantly melodic	11	1
Predominantly rhythmic	6	2
Melodic & rhythmic	22	5
Songs (text important)	7	–
Not specified	14	3
Global "specificity"		
"Specific"	17	
"Nonspecific"	17	
Not specified	49	
Presumed "specificity" concerning instruments		
Piano and organ	11	
String instruments	1	
Wing instruments	1	
"Jazz sound"	2	
Familiarity and/or "affective" content very important	15	
Novelty very important	1	

(with spontaneous *and* provoked seizures), at the beginning, the epilepsy manifested itself more often with spontaneous seizures than with musicogenic seizures. Females were slightly more often afflicted by musicogenic epilepsy than males. The first musically provoked seizure occurred relatively late (28.1 ± 9.8 years). In 78% of these patients with "musicogenic epilepsy" seizures were precipitated by hearing music, in 4% by specific sounds. Out of the 34 patients with a sufficiently detailed description, half had a very specific musical trigger, *i.e.* only a certain musical piece or a certain composer triggered the seizures. In the other half the type of music was nonspecific. In 18% (15/83 patients), the music precipitating the seizures had a strong biographical meaning for the patient. In only one patient, new and hitherto unknown music precipitated seizures. In 35/83 patients there were sufficient data on the musical interests and abilities of the patients *(Table III)*. There were 11% professional musicians, 31% amateur musicians, 14% "music fans", and 20% declared that they had a more than average interest in music. Although this might suggest that a higher "musical standard" may predispose for "musicogenic epilepsy", this question cannot definitively be answered since only insufficient data on the sociocultural background of these patients is available.

The pathogenesis of musicogenic seizures is unknown. With reference to the type of epilepsy, and the localisation and lateralisation, our review revealed the following: In 54 patients there were sufficiently precise data to allow the differentiation between temporal lobe epilepsy *versus* extratemporal epilepsy; temporal lobe epilepsies predominated (34 patients, compared to 20 patients with extratemporal focal epilepsies) and right hemispheric epileptogenicity was clearly more often reported *(Table IV)*. The suggestion of a right temporal predominance for musicogenic seizures is also supported by the documentation of right anterior and mesial hyperperfusion and right lateral midtemporal hypoperfusion at the height of a musically induced seizure during ictal SPECT (Wieser et al., 1997). This female (D.B. aged 32 years) suffered from right temporal lobe epilepsy. When confronted with her seizure precipitating musical stimulus, which consisted of Italian songs, she had psychomotor seizures originating in the right temporal region. At the beginning of such precipitated seizures she hallucinated "pleasant female murmuring voices, which progressively occupied her mind" before she lost consciousness. At the time we studied her with ictal SPECT and concomitant EEG monitoring she experienced up to one audiogenic seizure per week when exposed to this type of music.

A lateralisation of auditory experiential hallucinations evoked by electrical brain stimulation is also evident from the detailed study of Penfield and Perot (1963). In 520 epilepsy patients these authors have evoked — by intraoperative direct cortical electrical stimulation — auditory hallucinations 66 times in 24 patients: 17 times music, and 46 times the recollection of hearing voices. Music was evoked 13 times from the right hemisphere and four times from the left hemisphere. The sites of stimulation accompanied by recollection of music were temporal (anterior 5, middle 3, posterior 5) and opercular-insular (4).

In 1980 we described a young girl who had partial status epilepticus during presurgical depth electrode recording with prolonged right temporal discharges in the acoustic cortex that were accompanied by long-lasting musical hallucinations (Wieser, 1980). We then presented to her, who hallucinated a distinct song in her mother tongue, several types of acoustic stimuli including various types of music. Only with music that was very similar to that the patient hallucinated was it possible to document clear-cut changes in the epileptiform discharge in the right Heschl's gyrus. Our interpretation is that with adequate sensory stimulation it was possible to physiologically occupy Group II neurons, which without this acoustic stimulation were recruited into

Table III. Review Musicogenic Epilepsy (n 83; 76 patients from literature; 7 own observations): Musical Standard

	N 83	Patients with *exclusively* musically triggered seizures (n 14)	
Professional musician	4	–	
Amateur musician	11	3	} 15 } 27
Music fan	5	1	
Interested in music	7	4	} 12
Not interested in music	8	1	
Not stated and/or uncertain	48	5	

Table IV. Review Musicogenic Epilepsy (n 83; 76 patients from literature; 7 own observations): Localization & Lateralization

					Temporal*		Non-temp*		Clin	Seiz	EEG	Comb
					R	L	R	L				
Focal unilateral	35	Right 23	Left 9	Uncertain 3	18 (19) 24 (25)	6	5 (6) 8 (10)	3 (4)	1	3	4	24
Focal bilateral	19	R>L 4	L>R 8	Uncertain 7	3 (4) 8 (9)	5	1 (7) 4 (10)	3	–	–	3	9
	54	27	17	10	21 (23) 32 (34)	11	6 (13) 12 (20)	6 (7)				
Generalised: 2									–	1	–	1
									Some evidence by			
Not stated and/or uncertain: 27									1	5	–	4

Clin, clinical; Seiz, seizure; EEG, electroencephalography; Comb, combined evidence
* in brackets included are "uncertain" cases with some evidence

the pathological activity of the discharging Group I neurons. And that the sudden withdrawal of Group II neurons from the previously discharging "critical mass" prompted in the sudden change of the frequency and amplitude of the epileptiform discharge.

Zifkin and Zatorre (1998) found that more complex musical processing tasks activate more cortical and subcortical territories bilaterally, but with right hemisphere predominance. Thus these authors conclude that hyperexcitable cortical areas can be stimulated to different degrees and extents by different musical stimuli in patients sensitive to musical triggers.

Musicogenic seizures can be mistaken for nonepileptic events and monitoring may be needed to confirm the diagnosis. Patients may require medication appropriate for partial seizures. A unique very specific stimulus can be modified or avoided. The latency to seizure onset can also provide useful protection.

Comparison of EEG findings in musicogenic epilepsy and epilepsies with other complex triggers (primary reading epilepsy, language-induced epilepsy, and noogenic epilepsy)

Musicogenic epilepsy

As discussed, musicogenic seizures most often bear the characteristics of temporal lobe seizures with recruiting rhythms over one or both temporal areas, more often right than left. Figure 1 illustrates a patient evaluated with semi-invasive foramen ovale electrode recordings with a view towards surgery for refractory complex partial seizures of presumed mesial temporal lobe epilepsy. This middle-aged female patient, a high school teacher, claimed that listening to music triggered about 50% of her seizures. In fact, we could provoke seizures by having the patient listen to our previously designed musical consonance/dissonance test (Wieser & Mazzola, 1986). Most interestingly, the seizures precipitated by this musical consonance/dissonance test originated in the mesial temporal structures of the *right* hemisphere, whereas all her spontaneous seizures originated in the *left* mesial temporal lobe.

Primary reading epilepsy (PRE) and language-induced epilepsy

The EEG of PRE is characterized by evoked paroxysmal rhythmic theta activity or spikes either over one or both frontocentral, centroparietal or temporoparietal regions in association with jaw jerking. When activity is unilateral, the left side is more often involved, but bilateral jaw jerks are associated with this unilateral discharge. There may be bilateral or asymmetric myoclonic attacks and bilaterally synchronous spikes and waves. Studies of reading epilepsy suggest that increased task difficulty, complexity or duration increase the EEG abnormalities (Christie et al., 1988; Wolf et al., 1998).

Figures 2 and 3 illustrate the type of EEG that can be seen in language-induced epilepsy. The history of this 28-year-old male is the following: Polytoxicomania since 10 years (marihuana, ecstasy, cocaine, IV heroin) with some rare seizures in the last 10 years (no detailed description, about 10 *grand mal*). Reanimation after severe intoxication with Phenobarbital in November 2000. Incomplete partial transverse spinal cord injury, conus medullaris ischaemia with torpid paraparesis, and rhabdomyelysis with crush injury. Amputation of right leg. In January 2001 the patient reported myoclonic jerks when reading the newspaper. An EEG recorded on February 27, 2001 revealed epileptiform discharges provoked by reading and associated with myocloni and/or speech arrest. A video-EEG long-term monitoring confirmed such events with a very high frequency (480 times in 48 hours). Antiepileptic treatment was initiated with phenobarbital 100 mg/die and clobazam 10 mg/die and the situation improved, but reading still triggered epileptiform discharges associated with myoclonic jerks mainly in the jaw, associated with speech arrest or stuttering. These clinical signs and symptoms strictly coincided with the spike-wave or multiple spike-wave complexes, which were lateralised to the left anterior hemisphere.

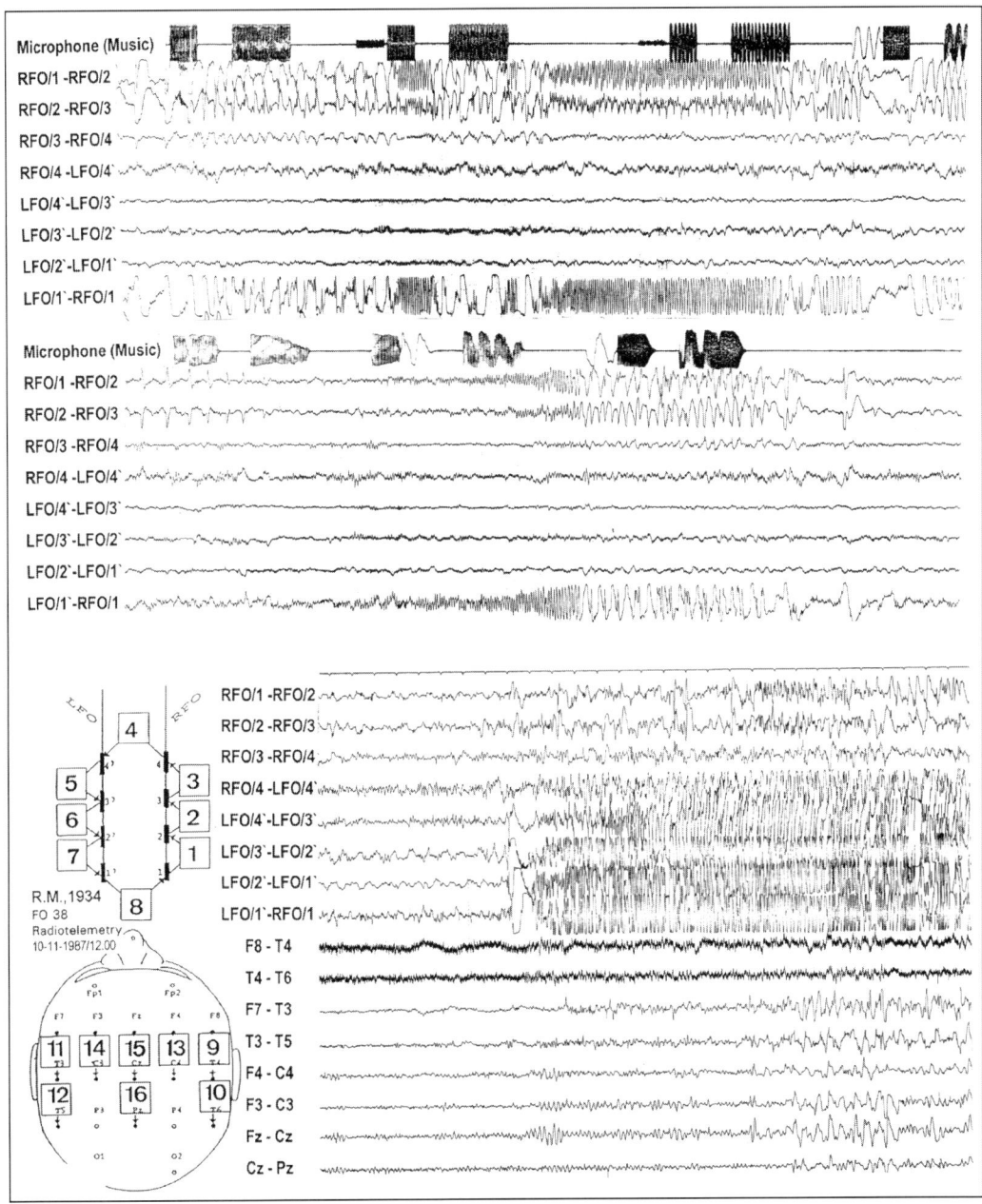

Figure 1. Complex partial seizures recorded with foramen ovale electrodes in a patient who claimed that about 50% of her seizures were precipitated by hearing a certain type of music. Two musically precipitated seizures are shown in the upper part of the figure. They originate at the posterior contact (contact 1) of the right foramen ovale electrode whereas all spontaneous seizures originated on the left (as illustrated at the bottom). The two seizures depicted at the top were precipitated by listening to a musical consonance/dissonance test, designed for another study (Wieser & Mazzola, 1986). The computer-designed consonances/dissonances were applied binaurally with earphones. The microphone signal was fed into the top EEG channel.

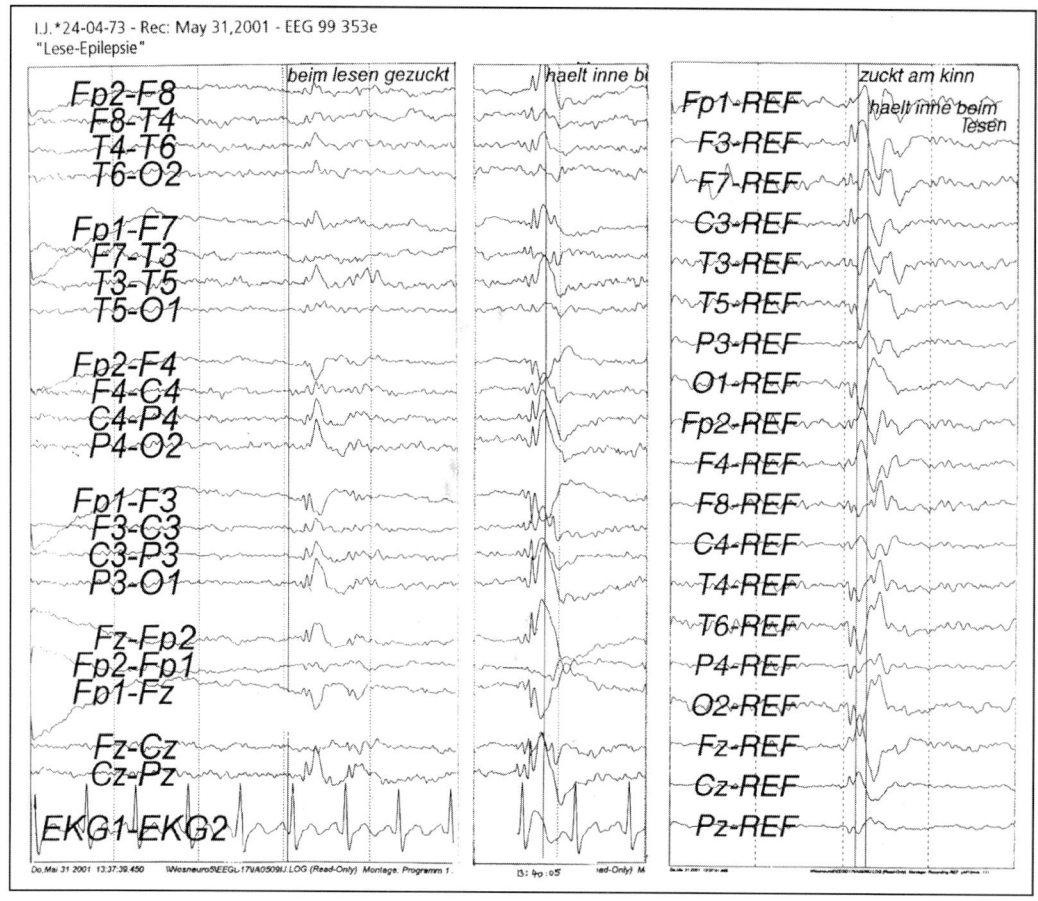

Figure 2. Three EEG sections with epileptiform discharges in a patient with symptomatic *grand mal* epilepsy who later on developed short seizures (speech arrest, jaw jerks) when reading (reading epilepsy). [EEG 99 353e. *24-04-73 May 31,2001]

Seizures induced by thinking

Seizures induced by thinking are typically associated with both spontaneous and evoked generalised bilaterally synchronous spike or multiple spike-and-wave complexes. Occasional patients have temporoparietal or frontal spontaneous EEG abnormalities. Clearly localised induced epileptiform activity is very unusual (Beaumanoir et al., 1989; Goossens et al., 1990; Andermann et al., 1998).

Musicogenic seizures and findings on the anatomy of musical perception 87

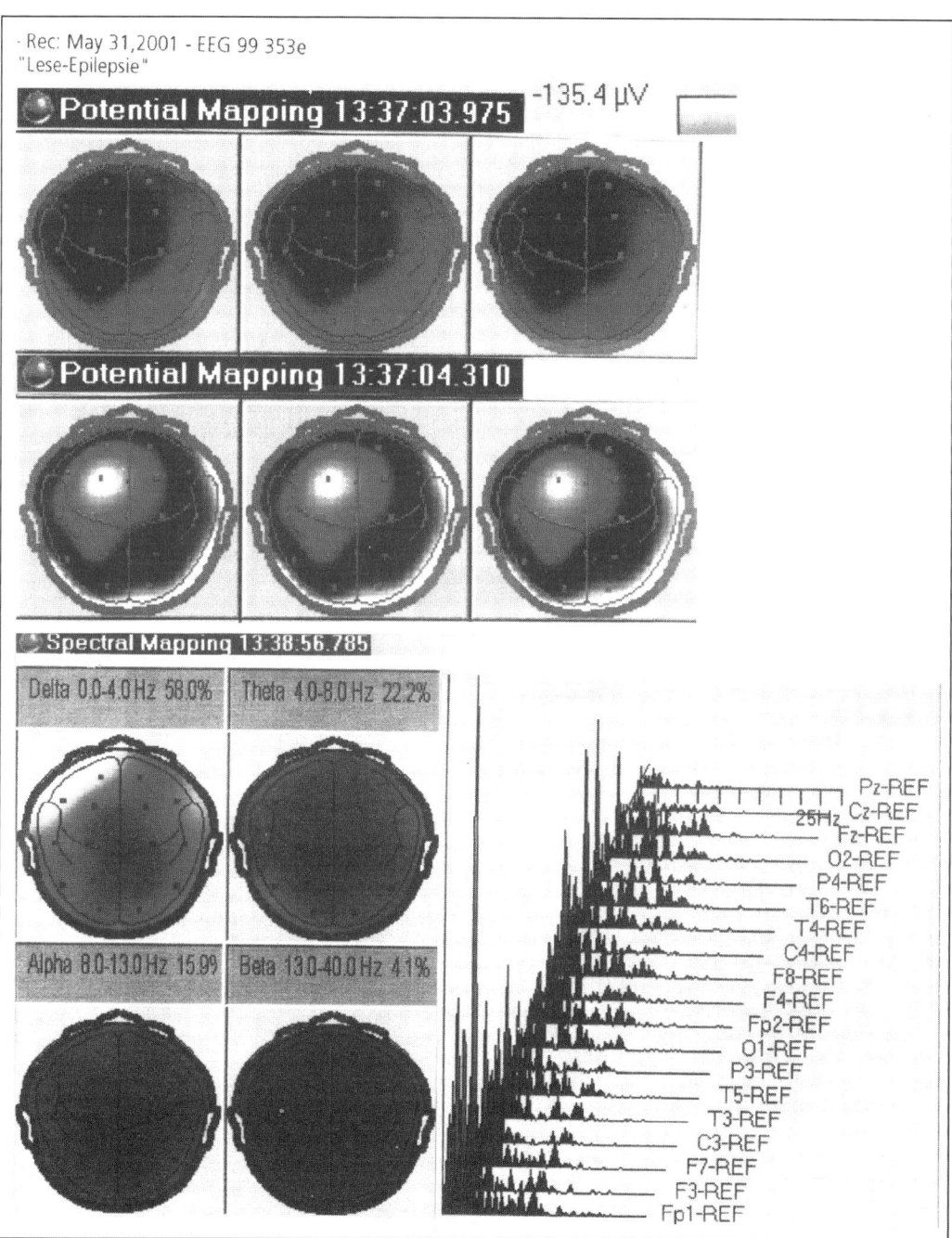

Figure 3. Potential mapping (upper part) of the initial electro-negative spike and following prominent electro-positive slow wave, depicted in *Figure 2* at right [myocloni of jaw, stops reading *("zuckt am Kinn, hält inne beim Lesen")* at time: 13:37:03.975 and 13:37:04.310] and spectral mapping with the power spectra (lower part at time: 13:38:56.758) showing a left anterior maximum of the epileptiform discharge as well as a delta maximum left frontal.

Findings concerning the functional anatomy of musical perception and their possible role in the ictogenesis of musicogenic seizures

We still know relatively little about the specific processing of complex auditory stimuli, in particular music, although impairments repeatedly have been described after left – as well as right – hemispheric lesions (*for reviews see* Benton, 1977; Dorgueuille, 1966; Marin, 1982; Zatorre, 1984). Most of these studies suggest that certain brain areas contribute in a specific manner. Today a variety of different techniques are available to study the issue of hemispheric dominance for auditory stimuli (*e.g.* monaural and dichotic listening, auditory evoked potential studies, scalp EEG analysis, neuropsychological task performances, as well as fMRI and PET). Dichotic listening studies in musicians (Gordon, 1970, 1975) and non-musicians (Peretz & Morais, 1979; Morais *et al.*, 1982) have found right hemisphere involvement in the perception of musical chords. Other studies, however, have found that both hemispheres are involved in listening to music, but suggested that differences exist depending on the individual's musical education, sociocultural background, etc., and in particular also depending on the internal "musical structure" of the tonal material presented (imaged and/or memorized).

In previous studies (Wieser & Mazzola, 1986; Mazzola *et al.*, 1989) we concentrated on the analysis of EEG changes in the limbic ("emotional") brain in response to listening to consonances or dissonances. We found that the EEG, recorded directly from the mesiobasal temporolimbic structures, reflected the consonance/dissonance dichotomy, whereas the simultaneously recorded EEG from the auditory cortices behaved differently. We therefore concluded that the limbic temporal lobe structures are important for the processing of music, in particular with a view towards the associated emotions.

In another study (Wieser & Wittlieb-Verpoort, 1995) we concentrated on the tone discrimination in patients with temporal lobe lesions and compared their performance with that of patients with frontal lesions and with controls. In a specifically designed tone discrimination task, the role of right temporal lobe lesions was tested for maintaining auditory nonverbal material (pure tones). Controls (n = 20) and patients (n = 52) with left or right mesiobasal or frontal lobe damage had to identify target tones in a series of target and distractor tones presented at random. Three levels of difficulty were defined for this task. Results of this study suggested a reduced storage capacity for tones and inefficient coding strategies for patients with right temporal lesions. Patients with right temporal lesions made significantly more errors than the other patient groups or controls.

While such studies may offer some insights into the processing of elaborate auditory stimuli and music, they offer little to understand reflex epilepsies and their mechanisms of seizure precipitation. The experimental focal seizure model of Wyler and Ward (1980) provides a theoretical basis for some possible mechanisms of seizure onset, which are particularly applicable to the triggering of reflex seizures. The model distinguishes intrinsically abnormal "Group I" epileptic neurons from instable "Group II" neurons. Using this model we tried to find some arguments for the notion that the precipitation of seizures by specific stimuli depends on the Group II neurons. It is our belief that specific seizure precipitating mechanisms and specific seizure preventing strategies share common features, insofar as both may act on these Group II neurons.

Indeed, in patients who had depth electrodes during presurgical evaluation with a view towards epilepsy surgery we had the opportunity to study the gradual transformation of normal evoked potentials following electrical brain stimulation to "giant evoked responses", to "paroxysmal evoked responses", and eventually to seizure discharges. We also could document the modification of seizure discharges by applying appropriate stimuli to physiologically occupy Group II neurons (Wieser, 1983; 1998). The gradual transformation of evoked responses to epileptic discharges may shed some light into the underlying mechanisms of transition from the interictal to the ictal state. It may suggest a gradual recruitment of neurons to the point that they reach a "critical mass".

An interesting model for the study of epileptiform discharge facilitating mechanisms is the application of weak DC magnetic fields. Prompted by the recent discovery of magnetite in human brain tissue we examined whether the application of weak DC magnetic fields could evoke epileptiform activity in epileptic patients suffering from the syndrome of drug-resistant mesial temporal lobe epilepsy. Candidates for epilepsy surgery who were evaluated by semi-invasive long-term EEG monitoring using foramen ovale electrodes were exposed to homogeneous DC magnetic fields in the order of 0.4 to a maximum strength of 1.8 mTesla. We found that in 4 of 10 patients epileptiform activity was activated by the magnetic field. Activation was most clearly evident in the 10-second interval following the application of the magnetic field (Dobson et al., 2000).

Finally the recently described "Partial epilepsy with auditory features" (Ottman et al., 1995; Winawer et al., 2000), a suggested autosomal dominant lateral temporal epilepsy, might offer some insights into genetically determined factors in auditory reflex epilepsy mechanisms. This syndrome typically begins in the second or third decade with infrequent partial seizures. Seizures are simple partial, complex partial or secondarily generalised attacks. A characteristic feature of autosomal dominant partial epilepsy with auditory features (ADPEAF) is that many family members report auditory hallucinations as their auras. These hallucinations include ringing, humming or machine-like noises or more complex phenomena such as distorted speech. Seizures are usually infrequent and response to therapy is good. Antecedent factors including febrile seizures are characteristically absent. Neurological examination, intellect and neuroimaging studies are normal. Interictal EEG studies are often normal but may show temporo-occipital epileptiform abnormalities. Inheritance of this syndrome is autosomal dominant with a penetrance of approximately 70%. Linkage to chromosome 10q has been found in some families, but the specific gene involved has not yet been identified.

Acknowledgement

I am indebted to Mrs. Simone Spring for help in writing this chapter.

References

1. Aird RB. The importance of seizure-inducing factors in the control of refractory forms of epilepsy. *Epilepsia* 1983; 24: 567-83.
2. Andermann F, Zifkin BG, Andermann E. Epilepsy induced by thinking and spatial tasks. *Adv Neurol* 1998; 75: 263-72.
3. Beaumanoir A, Gastaut H, Naquet R, eds. *Reflex seizures and reflex epilepsies*. Genève: Éditions Médecine et Hygiène, 1989.
4. Benton AL. The amusias. In: Critchley M, Henson RA, eds. *Music and the Brain*. London: Heinemann, 1977.
5. Christie S, Guberman A, Tansley BW, Couture M. Primary reading epilepsy: investigation of critical seizure-provoking stimuli. *Epilepsia* 1988; 29: 288-93.
6. Critchley M. Musicogenic epilepsy. *Brain* 1937; 60: 13-27.
7. Dobson J, St. Pierre T, Wieser HG, Fuller M. Changes in paroxysmal brainwave patterns of epileptics by weak-field magnetic stimulation. *Bioelectromagnetics* 2000; 21: 94-9.
8. Dorgueuille C. Introduction à l'étude des amusies. Unpublished doctoral dissertation. Faculté de Médecine de Paris, 1966.
9. Forster FM, Hansotia P, Cleeland CS, Ludwig A. A case of voice-induced epilepsy treated by conditioning. *Neurology* 1969; 19: 325-31.
10. Gastaut H. Synopsis and conclusions of the International Colloquium on Reflex Seizures and Epilepsies. In: Beaumanoir A, Gastaut H, Naquet R, eds. *Reflex seizures and reflex epilepsies*. Genève: Éditions Médecine & Hygiène, 1989; 181-91.
11. Goossens LA, Andermann F, Andermann E, Remillard GM. Reflex seizures induced by calculation, card or board games, and spatial tasks: a review of 25 patients and delineation of the epileptic syndrome. *Neurology* 1990; 40: 1171-6.
12. Gordon HW. Hemispheric asymmetries in the perception of musical chords. *Cortex* 1970; 6: 387-98.
13. Gordon HW. Hemispheric asymmetry and musical performance. *Science* 1975; 189: 68-9.
14. Hall M. *Synopsis of the spinal system*. London: J. Mallet, 1850; 100.
15. Marin OSM. Neurological aspects of music perception and performance. In: Deutsch D, ed. *The Psychology of Music*. New York: Academic Press, 1982.
16. Mazzola G, Wieser HG, Brunner V, Muzzulini D. A symmetry-oriented mathematical model of classical counterpoint and related neurological investigations by depth-EEG. *Computers and Mathematics* 1989; 17 (part 2): 539-94.
17. Morais J, Peretz I, Gudansky M, Guiard Y. Ear asymmetry for chord recognition in musicians and nonmusicians. *Neuropsychologia* 1982; 20: 251-4.
18. Ottman R, Risch N, Hauser WA, et al. Localization of a gene for partial epilepsy to chromosome 10q. *Nt Genet* 1995; 10: 56-60.
19. Penfield W, Perot P. The brain's record of auditory and visual experience: a final summary and discussion. *Brain* 1963; 86: 595-696.
20. Peretz I, Morais J. A left-ear advantage for chords in nonmusicians. *Perceptual and Motor Skills* 1979; 49: 957-8.
21. Ramani V. Audiogenic epilepsy induced by a specific television performer. *New Engl J Med* 1991; 325: 134-5.
22. Scott DF. Musicogenic epilepsy. (2) The later story: its relation to auditory hallucinatory phenomena. In: Critchley M, Henson RA, eds. *Music and the brain*. London: William Heinemann, 1977; 354-64.
23. Symonds C. Excitation and inhibition in epilepsy. 1959; *Brain* 82: 133.

24. Wieser HG. Temporal lobe or psychomotor status epilepticus. A case report. *Electroencephal Clin Neurophysiol* 1980; 48: 558-72.

25. Wieser, HG. Electroclinical features of the psychomotor seizure: A stereoelectroencephalographic study of ictal symptoms and chronotopographical seizure patterns including clinical effects of intracerebral stimulation. Stuttgart/London: Gustav Fischer/Butterworths, 1983.

26. Wieser HG. Seizure induction in reflex seizures and reflex epilepsy. In: Zifkin BG, Andermann F, Beaumanoir A, Rowan AJ, eds. *Advances in neurology*. Vol. 75. Philadelphia: Lippincott-Raven, 1998; 69-85.

27. Wieser HG, Mazzola G. Musical consonances and dissonances: are they distinguished independently by the right and left hippocampi? *Neuropsychologia* 1986; 24: 805-12.

28. Wieser HG, Walter R. Untroubled musical judgement of a performing organist during early epileptic seizure of the right temporal lobe. *Neuropsychologia* 1997; 35: 45-51.

29. Wieser HG, Wittlieb-Verpoort E. Tone discrimination in patients with temporal lobe lesions. In: Steinberg R, ed. *Music and the Mind Machine. The psychophysiology and psychopathology of the sense of music*. Berlin, Heidelberg, New York: Springer, 1995; 115-26.

30. Wieser HG, Hungerbuhler H, Siegel AM, Buck A. Musicogenic epilepsy: review of the literature and case report with ictal single photon emission computed tomography. *Epilepsia* 1997; 38: 200-7.

31. Winawer MR, Ottman R, Hauser A, Pedley T. Autosomal dominant partial epilepsy with auditory features: Defining the phenotype. *Neurology* 2000; 54: 2173-6.

32. Wolf P, Mayer T, Reker M. Reading epilepsy: Report of five new cases and further considerations on the pathophysiology. *Seizure* 1998; 7: 271-9.

33. Wyler AR, Ward AA Jr. Epileptic neurons. In: Lockard JS, Ward AA Jr, eds. *Epilepsy, a window to the brain mechanisms*. New York: Raven Press, 1980; 51-68.

34. Zatorre RJ. Musical perception and cerebral function: a critical review. *Music Perception* 1984; 2: 196-221.

35. Zifkin BG, Zatorre R. Musicogenic epilepsy. In: Zifkin BG *et al.*, eds. *Reflex epilepsies and reflex seizures, Advances in Neurology*. Philadelphia: Lippincott-Raven, 1998; 273-81.

Emotional seizure precipitation and psychogenic epileptic seizures

Martin Schöndienst

Epilepsy Centre Bethel, Bielefeld

▪ Introduction

To present an overview of research on the role of emotions in precipitating seizures is not an over-heavy task because very little literature is available. It is far less easy to design a scientific approach to studying the impact of affects or emotions on seizures, or, more generally, on epilepsy.

Though some clinical observations suggest that joy and well-being are highly effective antiepileptic factors, we know very little about how emotions and affects directly facilitate or impede seizures. Likewise, we know hardly anything about techniques for dealing adequately and professionally with affects when treating patients with epilepsy. Patients might also appreciate such knowledge as they often feel helpless when confronted with seizure-related affects, and these often raise fears in them, which may be so strong that they do not even want to talk about them.

This paper will first consider how affects have been treated in the development of epileptology. Next, some major methodological problems impeding an appropriate assessment of their impact on the precipitation of seizures will be discussed. This is followed by three case reports illustrating a few narrative characteristics that reveal the presence of seizure-precipitating affective factors in conversations.

We agree with Wannamaker and Booker's (1997, p. 1312) statement concerning emotional and other seizure-provocative factors that "clinical judgement is required to place the significance of this provocative factor in perspective for the individual patient". The goal of the present analysis, however, is to get beyond mere clinical judgements and demonstrate how the assessment of affects and emotions may decisively advance therapy by observing seemingly trivial remarks made by the patients, and the contextual gaps in their narratives with their consequences for the patient-physician dialogue.

The treatment of affects in epileptology

Since D. Janz' early article *Wut und Anfallsgeschehen* ("Rage and fits", 1947), there has been only a modest increase in our knowledge on the role of affects either as causes of epilepsies or as immediate triggers of single seizures. In general, during the decades since 1950, affects have attracted very little scientific attention. Disregard of seizure-provocative or triggering factors may well have been an inevitable consequence of a definition of epilepsies that specifically builds upon unprovoked seizures. But even at a time when interest in the precipitation of seizures increased, affective factors seem to have remained almost inaccessible to scientific investigation in the mainstream of an antisubjective and antimental, behaviouristically oriented psychology.

In many languages, terms like feeling, emotion, and affect have distinct meanings. However, clear demarcations are difficult, and will not be attempted here. Therefore, these terms will to some extent be used synonymously. However, it seems useful to distinguish affects, as complex total states in a person, composed of conscious and unconscious as well as mental and physical dimensions, from emotions, as perceptible cognitive aspects that become palpable to the person who experiences them. When affect is characterized as a border term between conscious and unconscious, physical and mental, intended and experienced, in other words, in terms of mutually relating dimensions, the definition given by Spinoza (1677/1985, S. 542), and still cited in the major physiology textbooks of the 19th century, has yet to be surpassed: "An affect that is called a passion of the mind is a confused idea by which the mind affirms of its body, or of some part of it, a greater or lesser force of existing than before, which, when it is given, determines the mind to think of this rather than that."

Perhaps it is this complex quality of affects or emotions, covering such varied dimensions of reality, which explains the wide range of judgements on their significance and effectiveness in life in general, and in epilepsies in particular. Whereas, for instance, Neugebauer et al. (1994) ascertained that "most seizures appear to occur spontaneously independent of any environmental precipitant or specific alterations of the body", Wannamaker and Booker (1997) proclaimed just as fundamentally the opposite: "in reality no seizures are truly spontaneous, as all result from the interaction of any number of intrinsic and external excitatory and inhibitory factors", before going on to underline this by stating that "most seizures occur randomly, but not spontaneously" (though perhaps what they really meant was that "most seizures occur unexpectedly, but not randomly").

These opposing statements indicate that the study of affects in seizures leads up to controversies that involve our ideas regarding the nature of seizures just as much as our practical approaches to treatment.

Freud, in *Dostoyevsky and Patricide*, was completely in step with contemporary opinion when he discriminated an organic from an affective epilepsy. He argued that "in the former case, mental life is subject to a disturbance from without that is alien to it; in the latter, the disturbance is an expression of the mental life itself" (GW XIV, p. 404, own translation).

In a paragraph entitled "Psychical Precipitation (affective epilepsy, psychic epilepsy)", Penfield (1954) also notes that "a purely emotional or psychological experience may likewise precipitate an epileptic seizure. The experience has in some way a facilitating influence upon the epileptic focus" (p. 39). It might have been this characteristic, comprehensive view of Penfield about the influence of emotional factors on a patient's vulnerability for epileptic seizures that made him insist that "one must treat the whole person. Most clinicians are convinced that the frequency and severity of attacks can be influenced favorably when emotional problems are properly handled. In special cases, analytical psychotherapy may prove of lasting benefit, but it should be used as an adjunct to anticonvulsant drug therapy" (p. 564).

Likewise, Hoff and Strotzka (1959) still took it for granted that epilepsies should be conceived as both "organic events for which a corresponding antiepileptic treatment is necessary" and as "mental events requiring a psychological therapy based on the techniques for resolving unconscious conflicts".

Particularly influential was Gastaut and Tassinari's (1966) statement in a paper on triggering mechanisms in epilepsy: "Emotions, according to certain authors, play an important role in the triggering of epileptic seizures and are even sometimes regarded as etiological factors of chronic epilepsy ('affect epilepsy'). We feel that this role should be most restricted, since we have been able to collect during our entire career as epileptologists only about ten patients whose seizures were regularly provoked by emotions. Furthermore, in none of these cases were we able to collect objective proof of the relation between the emotion and the seizure, a relation, which must be based exclusively on the say-so of the patients or their family." Although Gastaut and Tassinari do not go on to offer any data or references to support this view, their apodictic statement came to be cited broadly as if it were a confirmed fact.

Much attention has been given to a definition by Fenwick (1989) proposing that "psychogenic epileptic seizures" should be viewed as "those generated by an action of mind". He went on to discriminate: "Primary psychogenic epileptic seizures are produced by a deliberate mental attempt to induce a seizure" as opposed to "secondary psychogenic epileptic seizures... which occur when the subject is thinking, calculating or 'feeling', but not trying to induce a seizure". It is interesting to see how this conceptualization of psychogenic triggers focuses completely on conscious, rational, mental activities while broadly excluding affective factors (and completely excluding unconscious processes).

■ Methodological issues and approaches

As epileptologists, we are confronted repeatedly with indications that epileptic seizures may have affective triggers, but the mechanisms of such an affective precipitation of epileptic seizures are very difficult to investigate, not the least because affects are far harder to induce and operationalise during an EEG investigation than, for example, hyperventilation, intermittent lights or cognitive triggers.

Some major methodological problems for any scientific study of affects as seizure-precipitating factors include: How many affects can be distinguished? In what way can we observe affects, and how can we assess them? How much does the person having the affect feel it, and how much of it may only be felt by someone else?

Mattson (1991) reported a survey of 177 patients who were asked to estimate which factors triggered their seizures. The most frequent answer was "missed medication" (84%), which was followed by "emotional states" (58%), mostly of an unpleasant nature. In the same article, the author reported on an intensive monitoring setting to investigate a subgroup of five patients who "closely associated stress with seizure occurrence". He could demonstrate that latent hyperventilation, sleep disorders, and sporadic noncompliance are particularly important pathophysiological factors mediating between affects and seizures. However, the author was reluctant to more than speculate on whether "emotional stimuli can specifically trigger seizures by neural mechanisms".

Whereas Mattson's study assessed patients' self-reports, Webster and Mawer (1989) used a methodologically interesting approach to study the relation between seizure frequency and life events. They monitored 18 patients with epilepsy over a period of 1-6 years by compiling month-by-month seizure records and conducting interviews with the Life Experiences Survey (LES). The data analysis included two comparisons: (a) life-event months *versus* non-life-event months, and (b) seizure frequencies before *versus* after life events. Nonparametric tests revealed significant changes in seizure frequencies after so-called matched life events in 33% (n = 6) of their patients.

Temkin and Davis (1984) performed a statistically refined study on how self-reported "hassles" and pleasant "uplifts" in everyday life related to the individual probability of seizures over a 3-month period in 11 patients. They used the Cox Proportional Hazards Model to plot seizure occurrences as a nonhomogeneous Poisson distribution. Even after controlling for physiological precipitators, they still found a strong association with both daily stressful events and perceived stress levels in 58% of their patients. The authors concluded that their method of regression analysis could be applied as a flexible, individually adjustable screening in order to test whether patients are exposed to a specific seizure risk and, if yes, which stressors are involved. This recommendation seems to never have been taken up.

One aspect of Temkin and Davis's study is particularly relevant to the issue of emotional triggers addressed in this paper: they confirmed that emotional factors are not just able to trigger seizures as a direct temporal consequence, but that such stressors still retained a statistically significant impact on seizures after more than 24 hours.

Neugebauer *et al.* (1994) found a significant correlation (on the 5% level) between unpleasant events and increased seizure frequencies in 14% of 46 patients who completed daily questionnaires on life events and seizures over several months. Furthermore, they even noted the interesting fact that "protective effects of *unpleasant* events" could be found in two of their patients.

In summary, these findings contradict the widespread opinion represented by, for example, Troupin (1995) when he states that "popular speculation suggests that major emotional stress without other factors can cause seizure, but all evidence seems to be to the contrary. When compounded with sleep deprivation and perhaps problems with medication use, emotional stress of major dimensions can be an ancillary factor".

According to Wannamaker and Booker (1997) "emotional stress is ubiquitous and protean". And they go on to say that "evaluation for its presence should be a part of the initial assessment in every patient".

All studies quoted here strove towards reliable and scientifically valid knowledge on the basis of operationalised variables and the assessment of in some ways quantifiable and thus statistically comparable phenomena. However, to make subjectivity quantifiable, even if only partially, has a price: the variation from one person, and from one experience to another, is lost. For the sake of scientific rigor, specificity is abandoned in favour of generalisability. This virtually excludes from scientific investigation an important and complex feature of many seizures, *i.e.* the phenomenon first described by Pötzl and Pateiski (1937; 1957) using the term *Erregungsfang* ("capture of upset"). This referred to their observation that some patients in their auras would re-experience an important or traumatizing event of their personal history, which often was either related to the cause of their epilepsy or to the situation of their first seizure.

Similar observations, with the addition of findings with brain stimulation, became the basis for Penfield's concept of "experiential" auras (1954), which was later refined by Gloor (1990) who gives impressive examples of the affective quality of recollections elicited in experiential auras.

Feldmann and Paul (1976) reported a sophisticated way of using this phenomenon for therapy. In five of their patients, they explored the specific emotional triggers of their focal seizures. These triggers were then reconstructed in short videotape scenes for each individual patient. These "stressor tapes" were then played to the patients using a split-screen technique to record the scene together with an image of the patient watching it. Because the scenes triggered seizures, this produced recordings of seizures combined with their triggering stimuli. Repeated viewing of these recordings within a therapeutic setting led to a highly significant reduction in the frequency of seizures in all five patients. The authors attributed this to a learned ability "to associate the specific emotionally upsetting message input with the onset of a seizure", so that, once the patient "has acquired this information, ... [he or she] can consciously avoid the kinds of events which might be expected to induce a seizure".

■ Own investigations

Methodology

We have followed another approach, different again from standardized survey instruments, to the study of subjectivity and affect in relation to seizures (Wolf *et al.*, 2000). It aims at assessing subjectivity while retaining a solid degree of validity and reliability, and simultaneously takes a neurological-epileptological, and a speech– and discourse- oriented psychotherapeutic perspective. It focuses upon a structural linguistic analysis of the "say-so of the patients" (Gastaut & Tassinari, 1966) which has been shown to offer a decisively important source of knowledge because it provides access to the patients' "unedited" flow of thoughts (Drew et al., 2001; Peräkylä, 1997). In the spontaneous utterances of the patients, apparently unrelated ideas may supplement each other, and decisive clinical aspects can be reconstructed through an interactive, nonconfrontational dialogue between patient and physician.

The following three case reports will (a) present some special characteristics that need to be taken into account when assessing emotional precipitating factors, and (b) highlight aspects of treatment that may be derived from the identification of such factors.

Case Reports

Case 1

This 21-year-old male apprentice technician has a hypothalamic hamartoma and was referred to us with a diagnosis of gelastic, psychomotor, and *grand mal* seizures combined with suspected pseudo-epileptic seizures. After the patient's recovery from a coma induced by a suicidal overdose of antiepileptic drugs, a combined medicinal and psychotherapeutic treatment seemed appropriate.

The following presents a summary of his references to affective aspects of his seizures:

Patient: I have had seizures where I just screamed, was unconscious and bawling my head off and then I, uh, also <trembling voice> had stress and that has, I am certain, that has also contributed to me having seizures.

Doctor: Became stressed.

Patient: Yes, uh, I felt under pressure, have been, uh, also expecting very much of myself and when something didn't work out then I was disappointed in myself and I got seizures because of this. I screamed and the cleaning lady [who found the patient just after he had taken the overdose] *told me that I had been unconscious and lain there and had another seizure and shouted. Yes indeed, I was doing this apprenticeship and, and there it became after a while – it becomes more and more difficult and I also from myself... yes I didn't have any success anymore, the seizures accumulated.*

The parts of a transcribed conversation with the patient presented here were selected to demonstrate our method for analyzing the various subjective aspects of seizures, the psychophysical interactions involved, and the role of affects. In this interdisciplinary clinical-linguistic approach, first interviews with the patients are tape-recorded, transcribed, and then analysed in view of whether affects are addressed, what they are linked to, and in which patterns they are communicated. The ways in which we give each other insights into our emotional lives seem to be straightforward. However, our interview analysis shows that this can occur in two very distinct forms. In the first, less frequent form, affects are simply named as fear, joy, shame, or whatever; in the second, often ignored though far more frequent form, an affect is described indirectly via situational ("and then I ran away") or body-related indicators ("and then my heart was so loud I thought everybody could hear it"). The affect-focused analysis of 22 transcripts showed that epilepsy patients prefer to present their affects in a body-related or situational way, and one can regularly succeed in translating these indications into direct affect communications (Gülich & Schöndienst, 2002).

In contrast, patients with pseudo-epileptic seizures communicate the affects accompanying their seizures in a way that is often hard to decipher and full of contradictions – which correspondingly renders their translation more difficult. An example is a 48-year-old female architect who described her psychogenic nonepileptic seizures in the following way. Although it is very hard to translate a dissociated German speech in a way that approaches an authentic dissociated English, this will hopefully give some idea of what is meant:

Yes and then – then sometimes it's now never since its continuously in there is so for a few days is that never with the tension and cramps that's gone (4 s pause) yes and the other is a sort of second-long blackouts… no (5 s) prior feeling. Nothing. Nothing at all (7 s) yes and then like switching on and off (2 s) is that (7 s) then it was as if the – the light now slowly turns down like with a with the potentiometer and that is all like shifted into more gray tones and everything was a long way away and then just as if one is looking through binoculars like everything so closed in (4 s) yes then there was often also a sort of tingling involved.

Patient 1 is not presented because of the remarkable contrast between the seemingly cheerful appearance of his less serious gelastic seizures and the more serious psychomotor seizures characterized by impressive shouting. The focus is on what we so often unjustly found boring in our patient's repetitions. In contrast to what one might assume when listening only half-heartedly, for example, this patient does not simply report that his seizures are triggered by stress. By letting him carry on talking without interruption, and also paying particular attention to his repetitions within these interviews, or better still, referring to a transcript, one begins to notice that, like many other patients whom we have studied in this way, he repeatedly uses fixed patterns to address the specific trigger of his seizures. Examination of the short sequence quoted above reveals that the patient characterizes the stressor triggering his seizures in a very specific and idiosyncratic way: by repeating a specific combination of (a) stress in the sense of pressure to achieve, (b) an ego-syntonic achievement orientation, and (c) a strong fear of failure, he gives a precise description of his self-esteem conflict and how it induces his seizures. Almost as if he were testing this hypothesis, the physician proposed a corresponding description of the conflict in the interview. This had a bafflingly direct effect:

Doctor: Well, I get the impression that you had to fight hard for many years now against these constant restrictions…

Patient: [repeated, heavy breathing]

Doctor: [observing the onset of the seizure while simultaneously continuing his interpretation because the patient still seems to be receptive]… and also that you are fighting with a lot of energy, and that, so to speak, you are being really ambitious, with a lot of determination not to give up.

Patient: Yes. [*Laughs out loud, clear; first becomes louder, then lower, giggling; 16 s.*]

Doctor: And that is also – did this sensation rise up again right now? *(4 s)* mhmm, *(5 s)* hmm.

Case 2

The second patient, a well-dressed and charming young woman, attended our outpatient clinic for a single consultation in the company of her husband. This is a translation of part of the talk:

Well, I don't even know whether… I'll tell you what always happens to me; none of the doctors can tell me what it is… It all started after my daughter was born. The afterbirth didn't; it was terrible; they didn't tell me anything about how awful it was either, and the doctor as well, didn't tell me what he was doing; I felt like a carcass just lying on a slab; they tore out the afterbirth by hand. And then these seizures started; they always started at night; I always feel so nauseous, a tingling from my crotch up to my neck; you always have to keep on swallowing; it only lasts for two or three minutes, and then I always have to go to the toilet; now, it only happens about once a month; all of a sudden, body changes; you get headaches more often as well, and then you notice four weeks have gone by; you notice it's a feeling like a wave, like a birth pain; it's just, it's like you can't put it into words.

And, when it's daytime, I'm also aware of it all, nausea, this disgusting feeling, and this swallowing, I notice that as well; it then goes on for two days and nights; I have that a couple of times a day although I don't, don't think I do, lose consciousness.

At which point, her husband added: "I think the seizures vary in strength, but the type is actually always the same. The minor ones, they wake me up; she's breathing more heavily, and then I hear her swallowing and smacking her lips. And I put on the light and see how her eyes are open and staring. With the major ones, she sometimes doesn't react at all when I talk to her or shake her."

There is little doubt of a diagnosis of focal epilepsy: (a) abdominal and ascending aura; (b) constant semiology; (c) premenstrual periodicity; (d) occurrence of seizures in clusters that always start in night sleep; (e) oroalimentary automatisms; and (f) typical and constant duration of every seizure.

During the course of our conversation, the patient had a sudden *"flash"* that *"if I had had a chance to really tell that doctor what I think, the seizures wouldn't have been so bad"*. This led me to the idea that it might be prudent to try trauma therapy instead of pharmacotherapy – the normal indication.

A characteristic of traumatic emotional experiences is that they are not recalled or reported coherently but in fragments. The incoherence of the resulting narratives – which is often so irritating for a doctor seeking orderly diagnoses – is an important indicator for underlying traumatic experiences. Hence, trauma therapy essentially means to support a patient's effort to reconstruct and complete fragmented recollections. For the patient discussed above, treatment made numerous further details of the traumatic event accessible to consciousness. After initially triggering intensive affects, these then permitted a coherent recollection accompanied by freedom from seizures for what is now more than three years.

Case 3

This 26-year-old female office worker was referred with a tentative diagnosis of a dissociative disorder developing from previously diagnosed focal epilepsy with right hemisphere hippocampal atrophy. The patient reported:

It started when I was four years old. I must have been saying, "Mama, I feel strange", and I expect I was looking pale, so my mother took me on her lap. I suppose I was swallowing somehow, but it was always all over after two or three minutes. This even happened at night, as if it was only a dream, and then I would get up and go to my mother. And then, when I was twelve, suddenly everything changed. I didn't want comforting; I just wanted to get away. Since then, I always run away [author's remark: another physician had diagnosed fugues], *and I begin to scream, and they say that I make such strange gestures and I sort of swallow and spit.*

The patient is astonished by...

... a strange feeling beforehand, a feeling as if I have been in the same situation before. And, somehow, it's strange that it always happens in certain places: in the supermarket and, before that, mostly on the staircase at home. Sometimes I want the fit to happen, and I think of those places where it really takes place [primary psychogenic epileptic seizures following Fenwick's definition].

Two and a half years ago, it got really bad. After my aunt's death, I had two severe seizures in which I bit my tongue, and I was horribly stiff and aching afterwards.

In the further course of the history-taking, the patient described her early childhood as being overshadowed from the age of four by her mother's affair with...

... my father's former best friend. All I knew was that it had to be wrong, what was going on; but all my mother said was that I wasn't to tell anybody, and at school, I was always an outsider, perhaps because I was so full of shame.

Alongside these anamnestic details, the patient showed a remarkably unrestrained tendency to use all the available time to recount everyday occurrences, inducing an overwhelming feeling of tiredness in the therapist.

Whereas these observations might seem incidental from a strictly epileptological view, they are highly informative from a more comprehensive perspective. They suggest that her epilepsy is accompanied by an alexithymic disorder characterized by her failure to practice introspection, her inability to discriminate between affects, as well as her tendency to draw others into her isolation, exclusion of affects, and emptiness.

Ambulatory psychotherapy was started not with the aim or even hope of treating (curing) her seizures. Instead, we saw a need to foster a more mature self-reflection, counteract her depressive, in part, suicidal mentality, and work on the patient's exhaustive emptiness – what one could almost call her lack of access to her self. After a few therapy sessions, she surprised us with a completely unmediated cry: "*My mother and her lover could also have sat down and thought about where my seizures came from.*" Without any change in her antiepileptic medication (lamotrigine, blood level constantly below 1 µg/ml), her seizures disappeared completely after 15 sessions, and have not reoccurred during a two-year follow-up, whereas her longest seizure-free period over the last 21 years had been three months. It can be concluded that this treatment succeeded in curing her seizures, a treatment consisting of little other than a kind of retranslation of narratives back into emotions.

Discussion

In every one of these three case reports, affects play a different but, in each case, significant role in both the causation and the treatment of seizures. A therapy focusing on conflict of self-esteem is indicated and successful in the first patient. Trauma therapy proves to be a worthwhile approach in the second patient, and the third patient becomes seizure-free as a result of a therapy designed to improve her introspective and empathic skills.

Nonetheless, if the goal is to identify probable emotional precipitants of seizures, the preliminary impression gained from these cases may well be rather puzzling: in each patient, affects differ not only in kind but also in the way they emerge in the patient-physician dialogue. The first patient is able to tell us something about the hurtful impact of his unattainable personal goals on self-esteem, and even perceives some loose association with his seizures. The second patient has to deal with the enduring effect of a feeling of pain, horror, and rage focused on the person responsible for her trauma. The third patient, in contrast, is characteristically unable to engage in any introspection.

As different as the affects are in these patients, the important aspect is how each single patient manages to recognize the relation between his or her affects and seizures. The first patient repeatedly employs almost identical formulations to disclose an association between external pressure to achieve and an internal striving for success. This leads to an acute "narcissistic stress" that induces an immediate seizure. The second patient points only very hesitantly toward relations between seizures and her traumatic experience. It is only after much talk that she suddenly becomes able to forge a link between her trauma and her seizures. The third patient reports various aspects of her biography and the history of her epilepsy in a completely unrelated form. Only by gradually overcoming her affect isolation does it become possible for her to express the link between her specific childhood stress and her epilepsy.

In each of these patients, affects, epilepsy, and seizures reveal completely different constellations. Drawing on a traditional distinction in the modern philosophy of mind (e.g. Dretske, 1990), one could distinguish between triggering causes and structuring causes.

In the present context, triggering causes would be those that elicit seizures. Emotional triggers would be specifically those that precipitate emotional psychogenic epileptic seizures. In contrast, if an epilepsy as such has an affective causative factor, the affect would be a structuring cause.

In this sense, the repeated actualisation of the self-esteem conflict in the first patient represents the trigger for not only his gelastic but also his psychomotor seizures. In the second patient, the obstetric trauma forms a structuring cause for her epilepsy, and its processing with trauma therapy leads to the disappearance of her seizures. In the third patient, it is conspicuous that deficits in maternal affection and being forced to conceal her mother's adultery occur at the same time as the onset of her seizures. However, it is scarcely possible to confirm a structuring cause. Nonetheless, the provision of a therapeutic space in which she can practice finding her way back from narrative or scenarios to her affects and translating these into emotions provides the patient with an opportunity to overcome her specific inhibitions regarding intra- and interpsychological communication, and this is followed by a complete remission in her seizures.

According to Dretske (1989), causal explanations are context-sensitive. "What we pick out as the cause of an event depends on our interests, our purpose, and our prior knowledge." Nonetheless, it appears from the above that paying attention to affects in our history-taking of seizures is not just of academic interest, but also has important practical implications. As ubiquitous as affects are, they tend to escape the constraints of scientific rigor.

Our observations suggest the following recommendations:

1. One should not expect patients to offer the physician explicit links between affects and seizures, but trust that the cognitive unconsciousness of the patient will reveal them.

2. One should not try too rashly to link aspects of the course of illness to the patient's biography or personality.

3. Signs of affects take a variety of forms, and it often requires the interaction between the physician and the patient for them to become recognized and processed.

4. If the patient is given time to express him or herself, it is worth paying particular attention to repetitive formulations or patterns of discourse, to unexpected changes of topic, and to clues regarding what these patterns and abrupt changes relate to.

It is often the case the most important answers are not those given in reply to questions but those that are deduced from observation.

Final Comment

As suggested above, affects are complex psychophysiological responses to partially conscious, partially nonconscious internal and/or external challenges possessing a high intra-individual specificity. This makes them hard to access with a scientific approach in which the ability to isolate single, quantifiable phenomena is a decisive precondition. It would therefore be a mistake to conceive affects as being like easily definable stimuli such as flickering light, eyelid closure, startle, or even specific cognitive performances. Insofar, the present ideas on how to study, recognize, and perhaps even treat relations between affects, epilepsies, and seizures in the daily routines of the epileptologist may seem out of place in a book on reflex epilepsies. However, if we are able to go beyond our, at best, casuistic, but often only anecdotal knowledge on the pathogenic or ictogenic impact of affects in epilepsies and develop a methodologically rigorous assessment, we may find that some predominantly drug-resistant epilepsies become treatable when we process their underlying affects such as, in particular, shame, embarrassment, anxiety, and learned helplessness.

References

1. Dretske F. Mental Events as Structuring Causes. Lecture in the Conference "Mind and Brain – Perspectives in Theoretical Psychology and the Philosophy of the Mind". Centre for Interdisciplinary Research, University of Bielefeld. 1990.
2. Drew P, Chatwin J, Collins S. Conversation analysis. *Health Expect* 2001; 4: 58-70.
3. Feldman R, Paul N. Identity of Emotional Triggers in Epilepsy. *The Journal of Nervous and Mental Disease* 1976; 162: 345-53.
4. Fenwick P. Behavioural Treatment of Epilepsy. *International Review of Psychiatry* 1989; 1: 297-306.
5. Freud S. Dostojewski und die Vatertötung. In: *Gesammelte Werke*. Vol. 14. 1926; 399-418.
6. Gastaut H, Tassinari CA. Triggering Mechanisms in Epilepsy. The Electroclinical Point of View. *Epilepsia* 1966; 31, 85-138.
7. Gloor P. Experiential Phenomena of Temporal Lobe Epilepsy. *Brain* 1990; 113: 1673-94.
8. Gülich E, Schöndienst M, Surmann V (eds). Wie Anfälle zur Sprache kommen. Themenheft: *Psychotherapie und Sozialwissenschaft* 2002; 4/02, vol. 4.
9. Hoff H, Strotzka H. Psychotherapie bei der Epilepsie. In: *Handbuch der Neurosenlehre und Psychotherapie*. München/Berlin: Urban und Schwarzenberg Band IV, 1959; 646-59.
10. Janz D. Wut und Anfallsgeschehen. *Psyche* 1947; 2/1: 97-121.
11. Mattson R. Emotional Effects on Seizure Occurrence. In: Smith D, Treiman D, Trimble M, eds. *Advances in Neurology*. Vol. 55. New York: Raven Press, 1991; 453-60.
12. Neugebauer R, Paik M, Hauser A, Nadel E, Leppik J, Susser M. Stressful Life Events and Seizure Frequency in Patients with Epilepsy. *Epilepsia* 1994; 35: 336-43.
13. Penfield W, Jasper H. *Epilepsy and the Functional Anatomy of the Human Brain*. London: Churchill, 1954.
14. Peräkylä A. Validity and reliability in research based on tapes and transcripts. In: Siverman D, ed. *Qualitative analysis: Issues of theory and method*. London: Sage Publ., 1997/2003; 201-20.
15. Pötzl O. Z ges Neurol Psychiatr 159 (1937) quoted after Pateisky K: Die elektroenzephalographische Aktivierung bei Epilepsie unter Berücksichtigung von Mechanismen des Erregungsfanges. Wiener klin. Wschr 1957; 69, 713.
16. Spinoza, Baruch de. Ethics. In: Curley E, ed. *The Collected Works of Spinoza*. Princeton: Princeton University Press, 1677/1985; 542.
17. Temkin N, Davis G. Stress as a Risk Factor for Seizures Among Adults with Epilepsy. *Epilepsia* 1984; 25: 450-6.
18. Troupin A. Epilepsy With Generalized Tonic-Clonic Seizures. In: Wyllie E, ed. *The Treatment of Epilepsy: Principles and Practice*. Philadelphia, PA: Lea & Febiger, 1993.
19. Wannamaker BB, Booker H. Treatment of Provoked Seizures. In: Engel J, Pledley S, eds. *Epilepsy: A Comprehensive Textbook*. Philadelphia: Lippincott-Raven, 1997; 1311-6.
20. Webster A, Mower G. Seizure Frequency and Major Life Events in Epilepsy. *Epilepsia* 1989; 30: 162-7.
21. Wolf P, Schöndienst M, Gülich E. Experiential Auras. In: Lüders HO, Noachtars, eds. *Epileptic Seizures. Pathophysiology and Clinical Semiology*. New York, Edinbourg, London, Philadelphia: Churchill Livingstone, 2000; 336-48.

Trigger mechanisms in hot-water epilepsy*

P. Satishchandra[1], G.R. Ullal[3], S.K. Shankar[2]

MS. Ramaiah Medical college*, Bangalore, India
Department of Neurology[1] & Neuropathology[2], National Institute of Mental Health & Neuro Sciences (NIMHANS), Bangalore, India
[3] Department of Psychology, Mcmaster University, Hamilton, Ontario, Canada

Introduction

Reflex epileptic seizures are those that do not occur spontaneously, and certainly not unexpectedly but are regularly provoked by a precise triggering factor [1]. Since the time of Gastaut in the 1950s, reflex epilepsy has been considered as caused by preexisting cortical hyperexcitability, which upon a sensory stimulation produces paroxysmal EEG discharges accompanied or not by clinical manifestations. This cortical hyperexcitability or predisposition to epilepsy can be acquired or innate, and is most often genetic [2]. It may be localised or generalised. Generalised hyperexcitability may be intrinsically cortical or dependent on hyperexcitability of deeper structures. In humans, the stimulation best known to induce reflex seizures in predisposed subjects is intermittent light stimulation (ILS), whether by stroboscope, by patterns or by television. In humans, somatosensory stimulation may induce seizure manifestations without EEG expression.

Reflex epilepsies are interesting not merely as "collector's items" but provide extremely important information regarding the pathogenesis of epilepsy in general, and reflex epilepsy in particular. As the seizure-inducing mechanism rather than the etiology constitutes the common factor in these cases, the term "sensory precipitation of seizures" proposed by Penfield (1941) is probably more appropriate. Epilepsy with seizures precipitated by the stimulus of bathing with hot water pouring over the head is known as "hot-water epilepsy" (HWE) [3-9], alias "water-immersion epilepsy" [10] or "bathing epilepsy" [11, 12]. It was first reported in 1945 from New Zealand [13]. Following this, there were isolated case reports from all around the world: Australia [14], United States of America [15], Canada [10], United Kingdom [16] and Japan [17-19]. However, a large number of patients with this type of HWE have been reported from India [3-5, 7-9, 20]. A series consisting of no less than 279 cases of HWE, observed over four years (1980-1983) in NIMHANS, a tertiary care institution in Bangalore, South India, has been published [8]. A house-to-house survey – the Bangalore urban-rural neuroepidemiological survey (BURN) – of a population of 1,02,557 *(author: please check the number)* from South India, reported that HWE accounts for 6.9% of all epilepsies in this community giving a prevalence rate of 60 per 100,000 (Satishchandra *et al.*, unpublished). Mani *et al.* (1998) [21] published an epidemiological study from Yelandur, a rural area near Mysore (Karnataka), and reported a prevalence rate of 255/100,000 for HWE. The diagnostic manual proposed by the ILAE classification task force in 2001 includes hot-water epilepsy under reflex epilepsies [22].

■ Clinical features

Though it is customary practice among South Indians to bathe every day, washing of the head is done generally once in 3-15 days. The temperature of hot water used for bathing ranges between 40-50°C (the ambient room temperature is 25-30°C). Usually, in this part of the country, water is collected in a bucket and poured over the body or head using a mug. However, we have seen HWE in people using shower or tub bathing. This type of HWE has been reported in isolated cases from people having hot shower or tub bath from all over the world including USA, Canada, UK, Ireland, and Australia. Small series of HWE have been published from Japan and recently from Turkey [23]. Children are more frequently affected, although it has been reported in adults from South India [3-5, 8, 9]. In infants, there seems to exist a variety of hot water induced seizures where the patients respond to be lowered into the bathtub with their lower body parts (*see* Plouin & Vigevano, this volume). Males are affected more frequently than females (2-2.5: 1). In general, the frequency of the seizures depends upon the frequency of head bathing *(Table I)*. At a later stage in the natural history, 5%-10% of the patients manifest seizures even during body bath when water is not poured over the head. The seizures are complex partial with or without secondary generalisation. The onset includes a dazed look, sense of fear, irrelevant speech, visual and auditory hallucinations with complex automatisms. One-third of all reported cases have primarily generalised tonic-clonic seizures. These seizures have been witnessed in the laboratory and have been documented on video in some cases [6, 8, 15, 17]. About 10% of the patients express intense desire/pleasure and continue to pour hot water over the head until they lose consciousness which indicates the existence of self-induced HWE, similar to self-induced photosensitive epilepsy (Satishchandra *et al.*, unpublished observation). Usually, the seizures last 1-3 minutes, manifesting either at the beginning or at the end of the bath. A positive history of epilepsy among the family members has been reported in 7%-22.6% of cases. Spontaneous nonreflex seizures have been reported to occur a few years later in 16%-38% of patients [3-5, 8]. None had any neurological deficits.

Table I. Clinical features of published literature of hot-water epilepsy

Author name	Country	No. of cases	Sex M/F	Age of onset (years)	Seizure type	Temp of water in °C	Devt of nonreflex epilep. (%)
Allen	New Zealand	1	M	10	CPS	?	NO
Mofenson et al.	Ireland	1	M	7 m	GTCS	37-48	NO
Mani et al.	India	108	72:28	6-15	CPS, GTCS	40-50	16
Keipert	Australia	1	M	5 m	CPS	?	NO
Stensman & Ursing	USA	1	M	7 m	CPS	37.5	NO
Onuma	Japan	1	F	2	CPS	>39	NO
Subramanyam	India	26	58:42	3 m-35 y	CPS, GTCS	40-55	38
Parsonage et al.	UK	3	2:1	5.21	CPS	?	NO
Szymonowicz & Meloff	Canada	1	M	18 m	CPS	37-38	100
Itoh et al.	Japan	1	M	5.5	GTCS	39	NO
Kurata	Japan	12	1:2	5 m-9 y	GTCS/ATONIC	40-43	100
Miyo	Japan	3	2:1	3	GTCS	?	100
Satishchandra et al.	India	279	72:28	2 m-58 y	GTCS, CPS	40-50	25.4
Roos	USA	1	M	8 m	CPS	40	?
Shaw	UK	1	M	5 m	CPS	37	NO
Lenoir	Belgium	2	1:1	1	CPS	37	NO
Gururaj & Satishchandra	India	78	61:17	6 m-58 y	CPS, GTCS	40-50	12.8
Bebek et al.	Turkey	21	3.1	19 m-27 y	CPS, GTCS, SPS	?	62

m: month; y: year; CPS: Complex Partial Seizures; SPS: Simple Partial Seizures; GTCS: Generalised tonic-clonic seizures

■ Electroencephalography

Interictal scalp electroencephalography is usually normal. Fifteen to 20% may show diffuse abnormalities [3, 4, 7, 8]. Lateralised or localised spike discharges in the anterior temporal regions have been reported in a few isolated cases [6, 18, 19]. Ictal EEG recordings have obvious technical limitations and are difficult to obtain. However, there are seven published reports in the literature demonstrating ictal EEG recordings during provocation in water immersion epilepsy. They presented left temporal rhythmic delta activity [15], sharp and slow waves in the left hemisphere [16], bilateral spikes [19] and temporal pathological activity [11, 12]. Simultaneous split-screen video-EEG recording in one patient of "bathing epilepsy" had demonstrated delta waves starting from right hemisphere with rapid secondary generalisation [24, 25].

■ Trigger mechanisms

The exact pathogenesis of this unique form of reflex epilepsy is not known, but there are various hypotheses. Stensman and Ursing (1971) [15] suggested that these seizures are precipitated by complex stimuli, both tactile- and temperature-dependent. Though it was possible to provoke seizures in the laboratory by pouring hot water over the heads of the patients, similar stimuli such as hot water towels, sauna, or blowing hot air on the head failed to induce seizures. This suggests that the triggering stimulus is complex and may involve a combination of factors such as a) contact of scalp with hot water, b) temperature of water, c) a specific cortical area of stimulation, etc. Since complex partial seizures are the most common type of seizures, and ictal EEGs had demonstrated focal activity in the temporal or frontal lobe, Syzmonowicz and Meloff (1976) [6] suggested that there could be a structural lesion in the temporal lobe. However, CT/MRI done in patients with HWE have refuted the presence of any focal structural lesions. But even if such a lesion were present, it would still not be clear whether the ictogenic mechanism depends upon locally increased neuronal excitability in the lesions or, rather, upon pathological involvement of lower centres such as hypothalamus, or upon both [16]. Shankar and Satishchandra (1994) [26] have published autopsy findings in three of their hot-water epilepsy patients. All of them had spontaneous nonreflex seizures subsequent to the onset of HWE. The brains of three clinically confirmed patients with hot-water epilepsy (12 years, 23 years and 65 years of age) were studied. The duration of their epilepsies varied from one year in the first case to 15 years and 53 years in the other two. In the two adults, the disease process started clinically as reflex epilepsy, and later changed to nonreflex generalised seizures. The 23-year-old male at autopsy revealed a thalamic astrocytoma, evolving from low grade to high grade, and spreading to the temporal lobe, along with a wide area of subarachnoidal spread. There was no calcification. It is difficult to ascribe the seizure response to the neoplasm, though there is temporal lobe involvement. In the child, with duration of epilepsy of one year, a moderate degree of granular cell depletion in the dentate fascia, and loss of large neurons in zone CA_4 were seen. Zone CA_1 of the Ammon's horn on both sides had variable neuronal loss and reactive gliosis, on the right more than the left. In the 65-year-old male with a history of 53 years of seizure activity there was a moderate degree of neuronal loss in the dentate gyrus and Ammon's horn, and gliosis was noted, but less than in the subject with TLE of one-year duration. The patient succumbed to vertebrobasilar insufficiency. The pathological lesions in the hippocampus of the two adult patients with reflex epilepsy, when compared with epileptic lesions in adults with childhood febrile convulsions and nonreflex complex partial seizures, were similar on visual qualitative assessment. The neuronal loss and gliosis seen in the anterior hippocampus of these brains were similar to the ones described with chronic temporal lobe epilepsy [27]. This needs further validation by stringent quantitative evaluation.

HWE patients reported from India had a history suggestive of febrile convulsions prior to the development of this reflex epilepsy (11%-27%) [3, 4, 8]. This association between HWE and febrile convulsions has not been noted in other parts of the world. Febrile convulsions were found to be associated with complex partial seizures as an important risk factor in 20% of a population in a case-control study from Rochester, Minnesota [28]. Hence, the association between febrile convulsions and HWE is not higher than what one would expect by chance. The clinical behaviour of HWE patients during incidental febrile episodes with respect to susceptibility to seizure activity is still under investigation.

Experimental Animal Model

Repeated exposure of the head of adult rats to hot water (45°C) could induce experimental seizures, which is comparable to the phenomenon of kindling by repeated stimulation using subthreshold electrical current. Klauenberg and Sparber [29] called this "hyperthermic kindling". Satishchandra et al. [8] postulated that a similar phenomenon of *hyperthermic kindling* might be responsible for the development of HWE in humans. To further understand the pathophysiological and pharmacological mechanisms underlying this type of HWE, an experimental animal model mimicking HWE in its entirety – (a) precipitating stimulus, (b) the ictal events and (c) EEG comparable to those of human HWE – has been developed by Satishchandra et al. (1993) and Ullal et al. (1996) [30, 31]. A rapid rise in rectal temperature following a thermic stimulus in seizure-susceptible adult Wistar rats compared with seizure-resistant rats indicates a possible role of abnormal thermoregulatory centres in initiating the seizure discharge [31]. There could be constitutional genetic traits among the Wistar rats which make some animals seizure-resistant and others seizure-prone [32]. In the closely bred colony of Wistar rats studied, nearly 30% were resistant to seizure initiation. In the seizure-prone rats, the next progeny also revealed the susceptibility, highlighting a probable genetic basis. Following repeated seizure activity after hot water stimulation, the grey matter of cingulate gyrus and parieto-temporal cortex revealed shrinkage and atrophy of the pyramidal neurons, without gliosis. In the hippocampus, the neurons were depleted in addition to neuronal shrinkage and atrophy. Similarly, the granular cells of dentate gyrus also consistently revealed neuronal loss. Some of the neurons revealed apoptotic bodies. Reactive gliosis or microglial response was conspicuously absent. Some of the large reticular neurons of the brainstem, the Purkinje cells of cerebellum, and neurons in thalamus were shrunken and basophilic indicating anoxic damage. There was no evidence of focal myelin loss or oligodendroglial changes. In contrast, the brains of seizure-resistant rats and of controls not exposed to stimulation were essentially normal but for occasional anoxic neurons randomly distributed in the hippocampus and cerebral cortex.

■ Hyperthermic kindling in an animal model

Stimulating seizure-sensitive rats, seven times at a predetermined frequency of once in 2 to 4 days, followed by delayed 8th and 9th stimulation on days 15 and 30 after the 7th stimulus, resulted in progressive increase in seizure duration and severity, and decrease in rectal and hippocampal temperature threshold. This feature persisted subsequently even after 30 days, suggesting a phenomenon of "hyperthermic kindling" in these animals. Further on, the animals were sacrificed, and sodium sulfide perfused rat brains were stained by Timm's method to delineate sprouting of the mossy fibres following repeated stimulation. In the control animals, the Timm staining in the hippocampus was noted in the mossy fibre axons of dentate granular cells, which heavily innervate the hilus and extend into stratum lucidum of zone CA_3, ending at the CA_3-CA_2 border. In rats experiencing seizures following hot water stimulation, Timm silver staining was observed essentially in the internal and external molecular layer at the tips of the dentate gyrus, and the ventral and dorsal blades of the dentate gyrus. Following a single seizure, the rats sacrificed one day later demonstrated fine granular deposits at the tip of the dentate gyrus and the internal molecular layer. In rats which experienced multiple seizures and showed clinical and electrophysiological features of kindling, the silver staining density in the internal molecular layer at the tips and blades of the dentate gyrus were more extending to external molecular layer. Also in the stratum lacunosum, similar Timm positive reaction products were seen. Stratum lucidum of zone CA_3 had a dense cap of staining, which was minimal and focal in animals experiencing a single seizure only (Ullal et al., under publication).

The presence of sprouting in the rats in a graded way, highlighted by Timm's silver staining, indicates abortive reparative processes in the neurons leading to kindling. These hyperthermic seizures in animals could easily be blocked by using antiepileptic drugs such as Phenobarbital and benzodiazepine. However, phenytoin and the calcium channel blocker nifedipine did not block them [33].

A similar phenomenon has not been investigated in human autopsy material till now, though "kindling" has been suggested as the pathogenetic mechanism for progression over time of simple partial seizures induced by "hot water bath" to nonreflex seizures [7]. Further, translating this information to humans, Satishchandra et al. (1995) [34] have recorded the body temperature through a thermistor in the auditory canal in susceptible humans with HWE during hot water head baths. They demonstrated a "rapid spurt" in the temperature of 2-3°F within a short span of two minutes. Ten to 12 minutes elapsed before this temperature returned to baseline, once the bath was completed. This compares with a rise of 0.5-0.6° F in healthy volunteers, which return to the baseline immediately at the end of the bath. The finding suggests that this special form of induced hyperthermia could be responsible for causing HWE in susceptible individuals [31]. We propose that HWE patients probably 1) have an aberrant thermoregulatory system, and 2) are extremely sensitive to the rapid rise in temperature resulting during hot water head baths, and that these factors concur to precipitate seizures. The aberrant thermoregulation seems to be genetically determined. Further work to elucidate this hypothesis is in progress. The rat model described simulates human HWE and gives evidence that human HWE is a "hyperthermic" seizure [34].

Zenkler in 1960 [35] has discussed another concept of brain cooling mechanisms in humans. He has put forward the hypothesis that the cerebrospinal fluid may act as a temperature buffer for the CNS. According to Zenkler's anatomic explanation, dysfunction in any of the systems subserving this cooling mechanism could predispose susceptible patients to seizures in relation to increased temperature.

Since there are no structural changes in the MRI of humans with HWE, it is more likely that functional changes occurring in these susceptible humans induce seizures. To demonstrate this, we have recently conducted a study of interictal and ictal SPECT scans in ten patients with recurrent pure HWE after obtaining their written consent, using ethylene cysteine dimer (ECD). MRI, interictal scalp EEG, and interictal 99m SPECT scans were performed initially in these individuals using a single head scanner. Thereafter, the patients were stimulated with hot water head bath. Intravenous 99mTc ECD was administered to five patients (50%), who experienced HWE in the laboratory at the onset of the ictal event. The peri-ictal SPECT scans thus obtained were subtracted from corresponding interictal SPECT scans. Ictal hypermetabolic uptake was demonstrated in the medial temporal structures and hypothalamus, on the left in three and on the right in two patients, with spread to the opposite hemisphere. This preliminary SPECT study indicates the role of hypothalamus and medial temporal structures in triggering HWE [36].

Genetics of Hot-Water Epilepsy

Familial HWE cases with more than one affected member have been noted in 7%-15% of Indian patients [3-5, 8]. A single case of HWE in a monozygotic co-twin has been reported from Japan [37]. Among the 279 patients of HWE reported from South India, there were three dizygotic pairs of twins, each with one member affected [8]. From a descriptive epidemiological study conducted in the rural parts of Bangalore, South India, Gururaj and Satishchandra (1992) [20] have reported that 18% of their HWE patients had a positive family history.

Following the observation of induced hyperthermia, and the proposal of aberrant thermoregulation in the susceptible population, Satishchandra *et al.* have reviewed their cases for familial HWE and have found five families with two to three members manifesting HWE. It is interesting to note the co-existence of HWE and febrile convulsions in two of these five families [38]. The classic example of hyperthermic seizures are febrile convulsions. They affect 2%-5% of all children under the age of five years. They have a variety of causes, but a genetic component has long been recognized. Recently, a large family has been described from Australia in which febrile convulsions appear to result from autosomal dominant inheritance at a single major locus on chromosome 8Q13-21 [39].

The genetic mechanism underlying hot-water epilepsy in humans is not known. Studying the first five families closely, we proposed autosomal recessive mutation as a distinct possibility. We speculated that, although the frequency of such a mutation in a particular population would be fairly low, the high frequency of consanguineous marriages in many South Indian families could lead to marked increase in the appearance of HWE in this population [40]. The single locus model is, however, insufficient to explain any genetic linkage between these conditions. The influence of a modifier locus (or loci) or of environmental factors may need to be assumed to account for their co-occurrence [41]. Molecular genetic studies to unravel this are currently being undertaken.

■ Management

Earlier, hot-water epilepsy in humans was managed in two ways: 1) using lukewarm water for head bath or sponging with hot towels [3, 4] and 2) use of conventional antiepileptic drugs such as phenytoin or carbamazepine. Follow-up of 208 patients of HWE treated with conventional AEDs for a mean period of 14 (12.9 months (range 6 to 60 months) has shown that 60% could be easily controlled; of the remaining, 18.3% had 50% reduction in frequency. Others continued to have seizures at their last follow-up [8]. It is interesting to note that 10% of these HWE patients exhibit compulsive behaviour in the sense that they continue to pour hot water resulting in "self-induced hot-water epilepsy". Sixteen to 38% of subjects with HWE continue to get seizures even during regular baths and develop nonreflex seizures during follow-up (*Table I*). This is an indirect evidence for the phenomenon of "hyperthermic kindling" in humans, though the occurrence of kindling in humans is still controversial. In view of the observation that HWE is a type of hyperthermic seizure akin to febrile convulsions, Satishchandra and colleagues [42] have evolved a newer method of intermittent oral prophylaxis with benzodiazepine. They advocate the use of 5-10 mg of oral Clobazam 1.5 to 2 hours before head bath to be administered only on the days of head bath and *not* everyday. We have noticed that these patients do not require any other AEDs on a regular basis, thereby minimizing the cost and side effects of these antiepileptic drugs. Conventional AEDs are to be used only when the patients develop nonreflex seizures apart from HWE [42].

■ Conclusion

The development of an experimental animal model and careful analysis of human HWE patients have given new insights into the trigger mechanisms of this unique type of epilepsy, which can now be considered as a type of hyperthermic seizure. Aberrant thermoregulation in the genetically susceptible population with possible co-existing environmental influence could be the probable mechanism responsible for this epilepsy. Understanding that HWE is a hyperthermic seizure has led us to change the concept in the management of these patients from regular use of conventional AEDs to intermittent prophylaxis with benzodiazepines. Further, molecular genetic studies are in progress to isolate the gene responsible for this interesting type of epilepsy and to evaluate the role of canalopathies in hot-water epilepsy.

Acknowledgement

We sincerely thank M.V. Srinivasan and Mr. K. Bhaskar for their secretarial help in preparing this manuscript.

References

1. Gastaut H, Tassarini CA. Triggering mechanisms in epilepsy: the elecro-clinical point of view. *Epilepsia* 1966; 7: 85-138.
2. Naquet RC, Valin A. Experimental models of reflex epilepsy. In: Zifkin BG, Andermann F, Beaumanoir A, Rowan AJ, eds. *Reflex epilepsies and reflex seizures, Advances in Neurology. Vol. 75.* Philadelphia, Lippincott-Raven, 1998; 15-28.
3. Mani KS, Gopalakrishnan PN, Vyas JN, Pillai MS. Hot-water epilepsy – A peculiar type of reflex epilepsy, a preliminary report. *Neurology* (India) 1968; 16: 107-10.
4. Mani KS, Mani AJ, Ramesh CK. Hot-water epilepsy – A peculiar type of reflex epilepsy. Clinical and electroencephalographic features in 108 cases. *Trans Amer Neurol Assocn* 1975; 99: 224-6.
5. Subrahmanayam HS. Hot-water epilepsy. *Neurology* (India) 1972; 20 (suppl. II): 41-243.
6. Szymonowicz W, Meloff KL. Hot-water epilepsy. *Can J Neurol Sci* 1978; 5: 247-51.
7. Satishchandra P, Shivaramakrishna A, Kaliaperumal VG. Hot-water epilepsy – A variant of reflex epilepsy in parts of South India. *J Neurol* 1985; 232 (suppl.): 212.
8. Satishchandra P, Shivaramakrishna A, Kaliaperumal VG, Schoenberg BS. Hot-water epilepsy – A variant of reflex epilepsy in Southern India. *Epilepsia* 1988; 29: 52-6.
9. Velmurugendran CU. Reflex epilepsy. *J Neurol* 1985; 232 (suppl.): 212.
10. Mofenson HC, Weymuller CA, Greensher J. Epilepsy due to water immersion – An unusual case of reflex sensory epilepsy, *JAMA* 1965; 191: 600-1.
11. Shaw NJ, Livingston JH, Minns RA, Clarke M. Epilepsy precipitated by bathing. *Dev Med Child Neurol* 1988; 30: 108-11.
12. Lenoir P, Ranet J, Demeirleir L. Bathing-induced seizures. *Pediatr Neurol* 1989; 5: 124-5.
13. Allen IM. Observation on cases of reflex epilepsy. *Nz Med J* 1945; 44: 135-42.
14. Keipert JA. Epilepsy precipitated by bathing: water-immersion epilepsy. *Aust Paediatr J* 1969; 5: 244-7.
15. Stensman R, Ursing B. Epilepsy precipitated by hot-water immersion. *Neurology* 1971; 21: 559-62.
16. Parsonage MJ, Moran JH, Exley KA. "So-called water immersion epilepsy". Epileptology Proc 7th Internat Symp. on Epilepsy. Stuttgart, Thieme 1976; 50-60.
17. Kurata S. Epilepsy precipitated by bathing – A follow-up study. *Brain Dev* (Domestic ed.) 1979; 11: 400-5.
18. Miyao M, Tezuka M, Kuwajima K, Kamoshita S. Epilepsy induced by hot water immersion. *Brain Dev* 1982; 4: 158.
19. Morimoto T, Hayakawa T, Sugie H, Awaya Y, Fukuyama Y. Epileptic seizures precipitated by constant light, movement in daily life and hot water immersion. *Epilepsia* 1985; 26: 237-42.
20. Gururaj G, Satishchandra P. Correlates of hot-water epilepsy in Rural South India: A descriptive study. *Neuroepidemiology* 1992; 11: 173-9.
21. Mani KS, Rangan G, Srinivas HV, Kalyansundaram S, Narendran S, Reddy AK. The Yelandur study: A community based approach to epilepsy in rural south India. Epidemiological aspects. *Seizure* 1998; 7: 281-8.
22. Engel J Jr. A proposed diagnostic scheme for people with epileptic seizures and with epilepsy: Report of the ILAE task force on classification and terminology. *Epilepsia* 2001; 42: 1-8.

23. Bebek N, Gurses C, Gokyigit A, Baykan B, Ozkara C, Dervent A. Hot-Water Epilepsy: Clinical and electrophysiological findings based on 21 cases. *Epilepsia* 2001; 42: 1180-4.
24. Onuma T, Fukushima Y, Takeda T, Osawa T, Sato T. A case of epilepsy precipitated by hot-water immersion. *Clin Neurol* (Tokyo) 1972; 12: 386-93.
25. Roos RAC, Van Diyk JE. Reflex epilepsy induced by immersion in hot water. *Eur neurol* 1988; 28: 6-10.
26. Shankar SK, Satishchandra P. Autopsy study of brains in hot-water epilepsy. *Neurology* (India) 1994; 42: 56-7.
27. Rasmussen TB. Surgical treatment of Complex Partial Seizures – Results, lesions and problems. *Epilepsia* 1983; 24 (suppl.): 565-76.
28. Rocca WA, Sharbrough FW, Hauser WA, Annegers JF, Schoenberg BS. Risk factors for complex partial seizures: a population based case-control study. *Ann Neurol* 1987; 21: 22-31.
29. Klauenberg BJ, Sparber S. BA kindling like effect inducted by repeated exposure to heated water in rats. *Epilepsia* 1984; 25: 292-301.
30. Satishchandra P, Ullal GR, Shankar SK. Experimental animal model for hot-water epilepsy. *Epilepsia* 1993; 34 (suppl. 2): 101.
31. Ullal GR, Satishchandra P, Shankar SK. Hyperthermic seizures: an animal model for hot-water epilepsy. *Seizure* 1996(a); 221-8.
32. Ullal GR, Satishchandra P, Shankar SK. Seizure patterns, Hippocampal and Rectal temperature threshold with hyperthermic kindling in Rats on Hot-Water stimulation. *Epilepsia* 1995; 36 (suppl. 3): 552.
33. Ullal GR, Satishchandra P, Shankar SK. Effect of antiepileptic drugs and calcium channel blocker on hyperthermic seizures in Rats: animal model for hot-water epilepsy. *Indian J Physiol Pharmacol* 1990(b); 40: 303-8.
34. Satishchandra P, Ullal GR, Shankar SK. Newer insight into the complexity of hot-water epilepsy. *Epilepsia* 1995; 36 (suppl. 3): 206-7.
35. Zenkler W, Kabik S. Brain cooling in humans: anatomical considerations. *Anat Embryol* 1996; 193: 1-13.
36. Satishchandra P, Kallur KG, Jayakumar PN. Interictal and Ictal 99mTC ECD SPECT scan in hot-water epilepsy. *Epilepsia* 2001; 42 (suppl.): 158.
37. Itoh N, Kurita I, Konno K. A case of hot-water epilepsy in the monozygotic Co-twin. *Folia Psychiat Neurol* (Japan) 1979; 33: 329-30.
38. Satishchandra P, Ullal GR, Sinha A, Shankar SK. Pathophysiology and genetics of hot-water epilepsy. In: Berkovic SF, Genton P, Hirsch E, Picard F, eds. *Genetics of focal epilepsies*. London: John Libbey, 1999; 169-76.
39. Wallace RH, Berkovic SF, Howell RA, Southerland GR, Mulley JC. Suggestion of a major gene for familial febrile convulsions mapping to 8q;13-21. *J Med Genet* 1996; 33: 308-12.
40. Ramadevi AR, Rao NA, Bittles AH. Inbreeding in the State of Karnataka, South India. *Hum Herid* 1982; 32: 8-10.
41. Sinha A, Ullal GR, Shankar SK, Satishchandra P. Genetics of hot-water epilepsy: A preliminary analysis. *Curr Sci* 1999; 77: 1407-10.
42. Satishchandra P, Ullal GR, Shankar SK. Hot-Water Epilepsy. In: Zifkin BG, Andermann F, Beaumanoir A, Rowan AJ, eds. *Reflex epilepsies and reflex seizures, Advances in Neurology*. Vol. 75. Philadelphia: Lippincott-Raven, 1998; 283-94.

Reflex seizures in infancy

P. Plouin*, F. Vigevano**

* Hôpital Necker Enfants Malades, 149 rue de Sèvres, 75015 Paris
** Ospedale Bambino Gesù, Roma

Introduction

Reflex seizures in infancy are infrequent. Up to now, there is no reported syndrome in the International Classification of Epilepsies and Epileptic Syndromes characterized by reflex seizures only. In some syndromes, reflex seizures may be associated with spontaneous seizures, the type being the same or different.

On the other hand, seizures may be triggered by endogenous factors such as fever, but these are considered as occasional seizures and not reflex seizures.

In the literature one can find descriptions of an infantile form of hot-water epilepsy, a reflex form of benign myoclonic epilepsy of infancy, rare reported cases of photosensitivity e.g. in Dravet syndrome, seizures induced by eating, and self-induced reflex seizures.

Nonepileptic reflex seizures have also been reported and must then be differentiated from epileptic events.

Hot-water epilepsy in infancy

Cases of this type of reflex seizures have been described by Stensman and Ursing (1971, n = 1), Onuma et al. (1972, n = 1), Szymonowicz and Meloff (1978, n = 1), Roos and van Dijk (1988, n = 1), Shaw et al. (1988, n = 1), Fukuda et al. (1997, n = 3), Bourgeois (1999, n = 1) and Ioos et al. (1999, n = 4). Additional cases are included in a report of Oguni et al. (2001), on a group of 84 cases with severe myoclonic epilepsy in infants. The report of Bebek et al. (2001) on 21 patients with hot-water epilepsy combines all age groups. More recently (Argumosa et al., 2002) reported a new case that started presenting seizures when her head came into contact with hot water at the age of two months.

This condition is characterized by an onset of seizures before the age of one year. Seizures are always triggered by bath, immersion in hot water with a temperature around 37.5°C. When reported by parents they are described as "malaises", and when recorded they are typical temporal lobe complex partial seizures.

The neurological examination is always normal, with a good mental and motor development. There is no personal history and no family history of epilepsy. Interictal EEG is normal including sleep. CT scan and MRI are reported as normal, and no interictal or ictal SPECT has been done in these infants.

We report five cases referred to different children hospitals in Paris, four of them already published by Ioos et al., the fifth recently referred to us. In these five infants, seizures have been recorded by EEG or video-EEG (Table I). Immersion of the inferior part of the body in a bath at 37°C was the provoking factor. Seizures did not happen in cold water, and the colour of the bathtub had no influence on the occurrence.

Table I. Hot-water epilepsy, clinical and EEG correlates of the recorded seizures

	Semiology	Interictal EEG	Ictal EEG
Case 1	Pallor, cyanosis, staring	Normal	Left temporo-occipital spikes and waves
Case 2	Staring, chewing, apnoea	Normal	Left temporal spikes and waves
Case 3	Apnoea, hypotonia, staring	Normal	Right temporal theta
Case 4	Apnoea, hypotonia, staring	Normal	Right temporal spikes and waves
Case 5	Pallor, apnoea, jerks left hemiface	Normal	Right temporoparietal spikes and waves

In our cases, as well as in those reported by other authors, seizures had always a focal onset on the EEG, mostly on the temporal area (Table II). The semiology of the seizures could also be related to a temporal lobe onset. The outcome was always favourable when cessation of hot bathing was applied. Our five patients are free of seizures after more than three years of follow-up: no other type of seizure was reported, spontaneous either reflex or occasional. Fukuda reported the association with febrile seizures in his cases.

Table II. Ictal EEG in 7 infants with recorded seizures

Onuma, 1972, 2 years	Left hemisphere delta waves
Stensman, 1971, 7 months	Left frontotemporal delta waves
Roos 1988, 8 months	Right occipital delta waves
Shaw 1988, 5 months	Left hemisphere delta waves
Fukuda 1997, 6-12 months	1) Diffuse spikes 2) Diffuse spikes and waves 3) Diffuse spikes and waves

The differential diagnosis is often difficult. Gastro-oesophageal reflux may be associated with apparent life-threatening events mimicking complex partial seizures in infants, but these events have been rarely reported during bath. Syncope and aquagenic urticaria may be more difficult to differentiate.

From a clinical point of view, a correct diagnosis of this condition is very important. It is unproblematic to record an EEG when the baby is having a bath, so this has to be done. The treatment is very easy, *i.e.* to stop hot bathing. No AED is needed.

The mechanism responsible for this infantile hot-water epilepsy is not clear. It seems to be different from adult patients where the seizures are provoked by water falling on the head (see Satishchandra *et al.*, this volume). What is the precipitating factor: The tactile stimulus of the water immersion? The temperature stimulus? Is an additional visual stimulus involved such as light reflected by the surface of the bath, or the colour of the bathtub? These questions remain open as no model of immature animal with this type of epilepsy has been studied.

■ Reflex Myoclonic Startle Epilepsy in Infancy

In 1995, Ricci *et al.* reported a series of six infants with myoclonic jerks provoked by startle mostly induced by auditory stimuli. Two more cases have since been described by Cuvellier *et al.* (1997) and by Fernandez-Lorente *et al.* (1999).

In the report of Ricci *et al.*, there were four boys and two girls, neurologically normal, with a history of idiopathic generalised epilepsy in two cases, and febrile seizures in three cases. Seizure onset was always before the age of two years, and seizure remission was rapid with a total duration of 3-12 months (*Table III*).

Table III. Patients with RMEI, with family history

Patient	Family history	Onset	Remission	Duration
1/M	CAE	9 m	13 m	4 m
2/M	FS	8 m	12 m	4 m
3/F	GTC, JME	6 m	14 m	8 m
4/F	FS	12 m	24 m	12 m
5/M	FS	9 m	16 m	7 m
6/M	–	21 m	24 m	3 m

CAE: childhood absence epilepsy; FS: febrile seizures; GTC: generalised tonic-clonic seizures; JME: juvenile myoclonic epilepsy

Four out of the six patients presented spontaneous jerks associated with the provoked ones. One only had febrile seizures. Three patients received no treatment; VPA was prescribed for three infants, associated once with CLZ (*Table IV*).

Table IV. RMEI clinical outcome

Patient	Spontaneous jerks	Other seizures	Therapy	Follow-up
1	–	FC	–	3 y-1 m
2	–	–	–	2 y-1 m
3	+	–	CLZ VPA	1 y-5 m
4	+	–	VPA	1 y-2 m
5	+	–	–	11 m
6	+	–	VPA	8 m

The interictal EEG was normal in all patients during wakefulness as well as during sleep. Rare bursts of polyspikes and waves were recorded during NREM sleep. The ictal EEG showed generalised high-amplitude spikes and waves or polyspikes and waves, at 3 Hz, lasting 0.5-3 seconds, symmetric, with a frontocentral predominance. Deltoid surface EMG recorded brief rhythmic bursts. When jerks occurred during sleep, the EEG pattern was more irregular (*Figures 1-3*).

Clinically, the initial manifestation of the reflex myoclonic attack was a blink and 40-80 ms later the first myoclonic arm jerk occurred. The eye blink was not present when myoclonic jerks occurred during sleep. There was always a refractory period lasting from 20-30 ms to 1-2 minutes.

Surprise was a fundamental factor. Acoustic stimuli (both loud noises or soft brief noises) were efficient in all six children. Tactile stimuli were on the whole less effective, spraying of cool water on the face being the most effective variety. No effects of ILS or even single flashes were observed.

The differential diagnosis has to be made with other epilepsy syndromes with myoclonias during infancy, such as benign myoclonic epilepsy in infancy (BMEI) first described by Dravet *et al.* in 1982 which also occurs in normal children. The differences between the two syndromes are the provoking factors, the association of other seizures, the age of onset, the mean duration of the myoclonic jerks, and the familial epilepsy history (*Table V*).

Table V. Comparison between RMEI and BMEI

RMEI 10 cases	BMEI 40 cases
Provoking factors ++	–
No other seizures	Atonic seizures, falling attacks
Duration: 6 m	< 4 y-9 m
Earlier onset: 6 m	20 m
Shorter TT duration	Relapse of Sz
Genetic: 80%	31%
Male preponderance	*Idem*

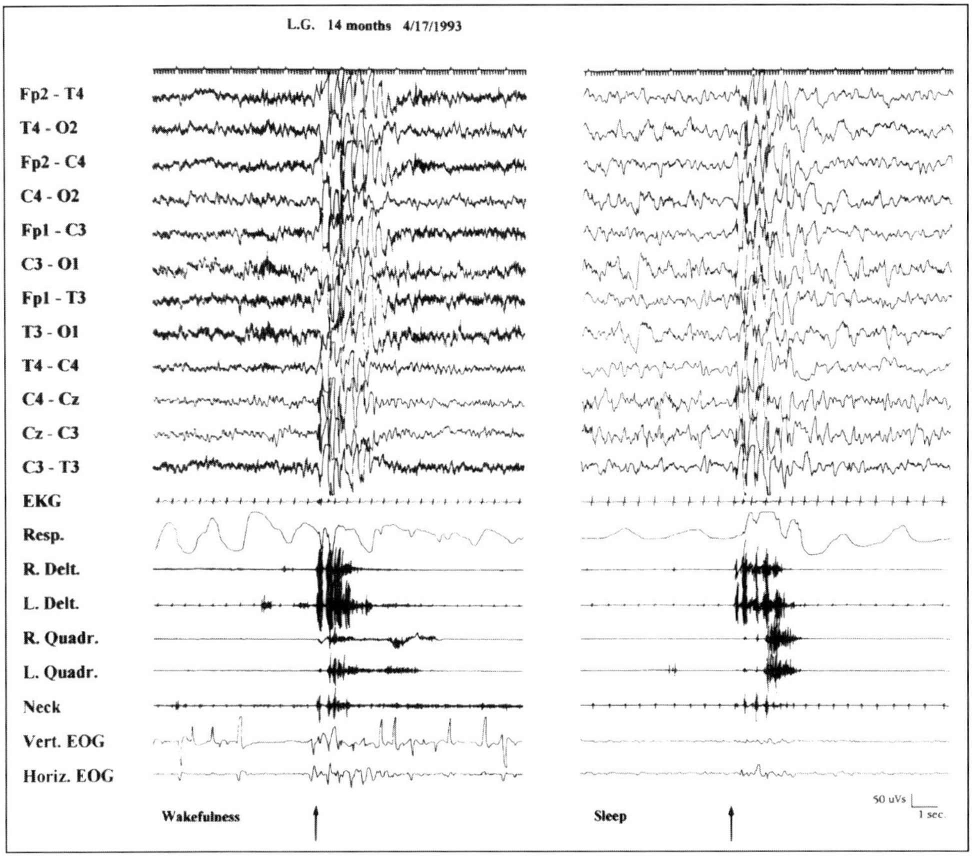

Figure 1. Patient L.G. with RMEI: two similar myoclonic seizures with spike and wave discharge in wake state and sleep, both triggered by a sudden noise. Arrows: stimulus.

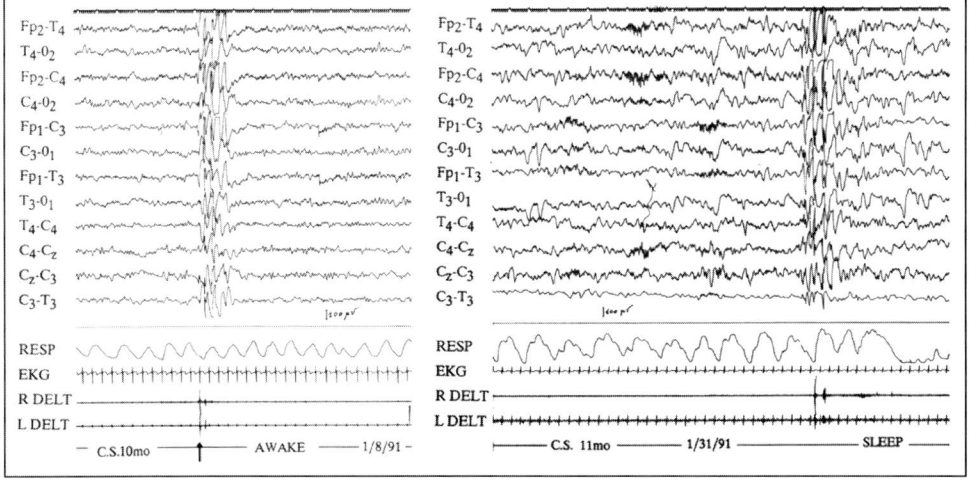

Figure 2. Patient C.S. with RMEI: a) provoked myoclonic seizure in wakefulness, b) similar spontaneous seizure in sleep.

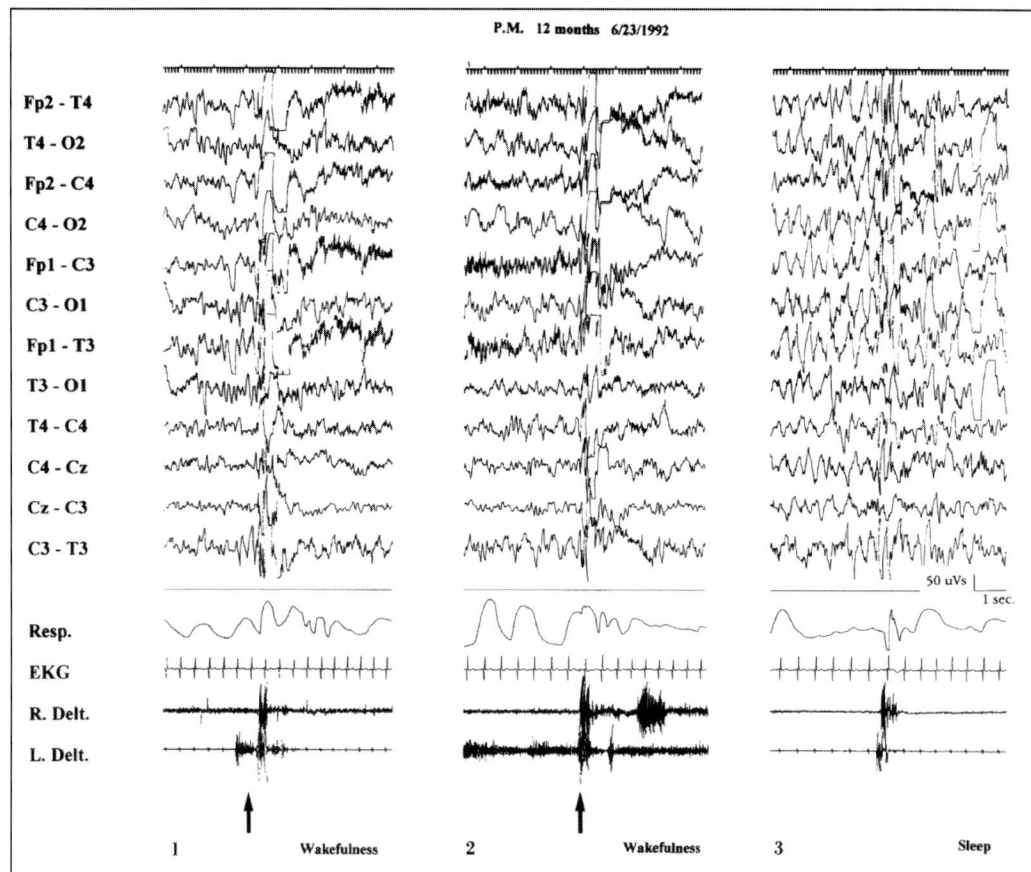

Figure 3. Patient P.M. with RMEI: provoked and unprovoked myoclonic seizures.

More recently Caraballo et al. (2003) reported eight children with RMEI, with the criteria of the patients first described by Ricci. No seizure was observed after rapid discontinuation of myoclonic jerks, with a median follow-up of six years.

The more common type of startle epilepsy concerns neurologically impaired children, but is very uncommon in young infants. Among nonepileptic responses with provoked myoclonias, hyperekplexia is one differential diagnosis to exclude: when the startle response is recorded it clearly appears that there is no EEG modification.

■ Other and miscellaneous

No photosensitive epilepsy is reported before the age of two years. In paediatric EEG laboratories, it is very rare to find a photosensitivity before the age of two, and never before one year. In Dravet syndrome ILS may be positive before the age of two years in 30% of cases but without clinical manifestations. Within the group of 84 patients with severe myoclonic epilepsy in infants, Oguni et al. (2001) found a subgroup in which myoclonic seizures and atypical absences could be triggered by constant light illumination, depending on the brightness of the light. This sensitivity tended to disappear before the age of five.

Only one case has been reported of an infant aged 15 months who experienced about 20 seizures in three weeks, when brought into a bathroom with bright white walls and shiny bright chromed plumbing: motion arrest, deviation of the head and eyes to the left of head and eyes to the left, jerks of the eyelids, looking afraid, and right occipital seizure on the EEG.

He had no seizure until 11 years, and again occipital seizures (Santanelli, 1989).

Eating seizures are infrequent during infancy. Navelet *et al.* (1989) reported four infants with the following characteristics: onset before six months, attacks provoked by meals, cyanosis, hypo- or hypertonia, apnoea followed by clonic movements of the limbs. A Gastro-oesophageal reflux (GOR) was present in the four cases. Attacks remained numerous although anti-GOR treatment was given and all infants developed a severe epilepsy. The first interictal EEG was normal and repeated polygraphic EEG recordings permitted to record the seizures. No efficacy of antireflux treatment on the seizures. What was the trigger: GOR, decrease of pH, pain?

Up to now the relationship between GOR, ALTE and epilepsy remains unclear.

Guerrini *et al.* (1990) highlighted that different types of reflex seizures are frequent in young children with Down syndrome and epilepsy.

Klass and Daly (1960) reported the unusual case of an infant who provoked seizure by looking at his own hand. Another instance of self-induced seizures is the case of a two-year-old boy described by Herskowitz *et al.* (1984) who provoked what seems to have been versive seizures by singing, reciting and using silly or witty language.

Leaving the realm of epilepsy, provocation of nonepileptic seizures has been reported in benign myoclonus of early infancy (by excitement or frustration, Pachatz *et al.*, 1999). Nonepileptic reflex seizures in the first months of life, triggered by passive movement or tactile stimulation when the child was held in a vertical position, was reported in 13 infants by Vigevano and Lispi (2001).

References

1. Andermann F, Keene DL, Andermann E, Quesney LF. Startle disease or hyperekplexia: further delineation of the syndrome. *Brain* 1980; 103: 985-7.
2. Argumosa A, Herranz JL, Barrasa J, Arteaga R. Reflex epilepsy from hot water: a new case and review of the literature. *Rev Neurol* 2002; 35: 349-53.
3. Bebek N, Gürses C, Gokyigit A, Baykan B, Özkara C, Dervent A. Hot-water epilepsy: clinical and electrophysiologic findings based on 21 cases. *Epilepsia* 2001; 42: 1180-4.
4. Bourgeois BF. A retarded boy with seizures precipitated by stepping into the bath water. *Semin Pediatr Neurol* 1999; 6: 156-7.

5. Caraballo R, Casar L, Monges S, Yepez I, Galicchio S, Cersosimo R, Fejerman N. Reflex myoclonic epilepsy in infancy: a new reflex epilepsy syndrome or a variant of benign myoclonic epilepsy in infancy. *Rev Neurol* 2003; 36: 429-32.
6. Cuvellier JC, Lamblin MD, Cuisset JM, Vallée L, Nuyts JP. Benign reflex myoclonic epilepsy in infancy. *Arch Pediatr* 1997; 4: 755-8.
7. Dravet C, Bureau M, Roger J. Benign myoclonic epilepsy in infants. In: Roger J, Bureau M, Dravet C, Dreifuss FE, Perret J, Wolf P, eds. *Epileptic syndromes in infancy, childhood and adolescence*, 2nd ed. London, Paris: John Libbey, 1992: 67-74.
8. Fernandez-Lorente J, Pastor J, Carbonell J, Aparicio-Meix JM. Reflex benign myoclonic epilepsy of childhood. Apropos of a new case. *Rev neurol* 1999; 29: 39-42.
9. Fukuda M, Morimoto T, Nagao H, Kida K. Clinical study of epilepsy with severe febrile seizures and seizures induced by hot water. *Brain and Dev* 1997; 19: 212-6.
10. Guerrini R, Genton P, Bureau M, Dravet C, Roger J. Reflex seizures are frequent in patients with Down syndrome and epilepsy. *Epilepsia* 1990; 31: 406-17.
11. Herskowitz J, Rosman NP, Geschwind N. Seizures induced by singing and recitation. A unique form of reflex epilepsy in childhood. *Arch Neurol* 1984; 41: 1102-3.
12. Ioos C, Villeneuve N, Fohlen M, Badinant-Hubert N, Jalin C, Cheliout-Heraut F, Pinard JM. Hot-water epilepsy: a benign and underestimated form. *Arch Pediatr* 1999; 6: 755-8.
13. Klass DW, Daly DD. An unusual seizure induction mechanism ("manugenic"). *Electroencephal Clin Neurophysiol* 1960; 12: 156.
14. Oguni H, Hayashi K, Awaya Y, Fukuyama Y, Osawa M. Severe myoclonic epilepsy in infants – a review based on the Tokyo Women's Medical University series of 84 cases. *Brain Dev* 2001; 23: 736-48.
15. Onuma T, Fukushima Y, Tallada T. A case of epilepsy precipitated by hot water immersion. *Clin Neurol* (Tokyo) 1972; 12: 386-93.
16. Pachatz C, Fusco L, Vigevano F. Benign myoclonus of early infancy. *Epileptic Disord* 1999; 1: 57-61.
17. Ricci S, Cusmai R, Fusco L, Vigevano F. Reflex myoclonic epilepsy in infancy: a new age-dependent idiopathic epilepsy syndrome related to startle reaction. *Epilepsia* 1995; 36: 342-8.
18. Roos RA, van Dijk JG. Reflex epilepsy induced by immersion in hot water. *Europ Neurol* 1988; 28: 6-10.
19. Santanelli P, Mancini J, Gastaut H. An electroencephalographic demonstration of auricular reflex epilepsy. *Epilepsia* 1985; 26: 95-7.
20. Shaw NJ, Livingston JH, Minns RA, Clarke M. Epilepsy precipitated by bathing. *Dev Med Child Neurol* 1988; 30: 108-11.
21. Stensman R, Ursing B. Epilepsy precipitated by (bathing) hot water immersion. *Neurology* 1971; 21: 559-62.
22. Szymonowicz W, Meloff KL. Hot-water epilepsy. *Can J Neurol Sci* 1978; 2: 247-51.
23. Vigevano F, Lispi ML. Tonic reflex seizures of early infancy: an age-related nonepileptic paroxysmal disorder. *Epileptic Disord* 2001; 3: 133-6.

Seizures induced by eating in a family

E.M.T. Yacubian, R. Skaff, E. Garzon, N.I.O. Braga, A.C. Sakamoto, H. Carrete

Department of Neurology, Escola Paulista de Medicina, Universidade Federal de São Paulo. Centro de Epilepsia do Hospital Alemão Oswaldo Cruz, São Paulo, Brazil

■ Summary

Eating seizures with probable temporolimbic onset were observed in three women of eight individuals from the same family with epilepsy. The epilepsy onset was in the second decade of life in all cases and the seizures were characterized by staring, oroalimentary automatisms, and alteration of consciousness followed by motor signs. All patients presented relatively frequent seizures, most of them induced by eating. Seizures recorded while eating showed diffuse abnormalities. Antiepileptic drugs could not lead to complete control of the seizures. High-resolution MRI emphasizing the temporal lobe structures and perisylvian regions did not show any abnormality. Temporal lobe epilepsy with seizures not related to eating and myoclonic juvenile epilepsy were present in other family members. In this family, despite the difficulty in seizure control and the high seizure frequency, eating temporolimbic seizures may represent a manifestation of an idiopathic form of temporal lobe epilepsy.

■ Introduction

Seizures induced by eating are usually seen in symptomatic localisation-related epilepsies. Although some patients with idiopathic generalised epilepsies have been reported, they are considered exceptional and not well documented (Zifkin *et al.*, 1994). Eating epilepsy, as defined by Rémillard *et al.* in 1989, has been classified into two distinct groups, with either a temporal or a perisylvian seizure onset. Temporolimbic onset is the most common presentation of this rare type of epilepsy being responsible for approximately 70% of the cases. Among the temporolimbic structures, it has been suggested that the amygdala very likely plays an important role in eating seizures because of its low threshold for seizure activity and its involvement in masticatory movements (Ahuja et al., 1980; Reder & Wright, 1982).

Senanayake (1990a) first described familial eating epilepsy in 20 out of 59 siblings from nine different families residing in Sri Lanka. The epilepsy was characterized by partial seizures in all the 20 patients being complex partial in 15 and simple partial in five. This author emphasized the tendency of secondary generalisation of the partial seizures in these patients. On the other hand, familial temporal lobe epilepsy has only recently been described in the literature. The first series described familial temporal lobe epilepsy as a benign disorder in which the affected individuals had a homogeneous pattern of temporal lobe epilepsy, with late onset of seizures and good outcome. MRI was normal and the EEG showed sparse temporal interictal epileptiform discharges in only 22% of subjects (Berkovic et al., 1994). A second report of familial temporal lobe epilepsy identified 36 affected individuals in 11 unrelated families with clinical heterogeneity. Although the majority of these patients presented good seizure control, some of them had intractable epilepsy and required surgical treatment. MRI was available in 18 subjects and showed features of mesial temporal sclerosis in 11 (61%) of them (Cendes et al., 1998). More recently, a larger series analyzing 98 individuals with seizures from 22 unrelated families was published (Kobayashi et al., 2001). This series confirmed the heterogeneity of familial temporal lobe epilepsy and described hippocampal atrophy in 57% of the patients, including those with benign course or seizure remission.

Idiopathic familial focal epilepsies with seizures induced by eating have only been described in families from Sri Lanka (Senanayake, 1990a). We describe a Brazilian family in which possible temporolimbic seizures induced by eating were diagnosed in three of its eight members with epilepsy.

■ Case reports

A 23-year-old female presented seizure onset at 16. There were no important antecedents in her personal history. Her seizures were almost always related to regular meals and characterized by a suffocating feeling, a tightness over the chest and an assurance that something was about to happen. These sensations were followed by a warning of loss of consciousness during which she felt that she would be able to preview what was going to happen in the future for a few seconds. After impairment of consciousness she presented staring, oroalimentary and right arm automatisms during which she repeatedly fiddled with the cutlery. These episodes were short and followed by a slight confusion. Sometimes she presented seizures with initial loss of consciousness. As her seizures were related to eating, and in order to prevent having them when with fellow workers, she avoided having lunch when at work. Rarely, seizures with the same symptomatology occurred spontaneously. She also presented secondary generalised seizures during sleep. In the beginning she used to have five seizures per week, and nowadays she is having only seizures related to meals at a frequency of about 1/month. Phenobarbital (300 mg/day) could not significantly modify the seizure frequency and carbamazepine (up to 1000 mg/day), her present medication, improved the seizure frequency. She denied complaints about memory. The video-EEG recording showed rare sharp waves occurring independently over the temporal lobe leads most predominantly in the right sphenoidal and in T7. A seizure recorded during dinner is showed in *Figures 1a* and *1b*. The video analysis showed that after having received the meal on a tray she started to fiddle with the utensils used for serving, in order to unwrap them. It took her seven minutes to do this without feeding herself. Intermittent diffuse long runs of theta activity mainly over the anterior areas of both cerebral hemispheres appeared on EEG waxing and waning all this time (*Figure 1a*). This activity completely disappeared when she had to attend a telephone call and spoke for about 1.5 minutes. Soon after hanging up she took the first helping of food to the mouth and started masticating. Suddenly thereafter, she stopped eating and presented staring, became irresponsive, continued chewing and moving the fork on the right automatically and presented a change in heart frequency from 84 to 114. The duration of the seizure was 90 seconds and at the time of the clinical seizure onset the EEG showed an abrupt interruption of the theta runs which were substituted by a low voltage EEG till the end of the seizure (*Figure 1b*). The high-resolution MRI, emphasizing the temporal lobe structures, was normal (*Figure 2*).

Her 18-year-old sister hadn't present important factors in her past history either. She had had seizures since 12, when she presented a complex partial seizure during sleep. Some months later she started presenting complex partial seizures mostly at breakfast. At present, about 70% of the episodes have been related to eating and not to a specific kind of food or drink. These episodes were characterized by staring, irresponsiveness, oroalimentary and manual automatisms followed by eyes and head turning to the right. At the end of the seizures she presents difficulty in pronunciation of words. The seizure frequency was about 3/week. Secondary generalisation could rarely occur (since the beginning of the epilepsy she presented only seven generalised tonic-clonic seizures). Phenobarbital (150 mg/day) did not change the seizure frequency while carbamazepine (600 mg/day) improved the seizure control. The video-EEG revealed frequent bursts of regular spike-wave complexes activated by hyperventilation and generalised polyspike discharges during sleep, when some sharp waves also appeared over the posterior temporal regions (*Figures 3* and *4*). One seizure was recorded while having lunch. This was a complete and prolonged meal, which involved food, juice and dessert. Approximately 47 minutes had gone by when she was having a bar of chocolate; she suddenly dropped it and presented behavioural arrest, staring, and oculocephalic version to the right, oroalimentary automatisms and right arm dystonic posturing. The seizure lasted one minute and mental confusion, somnolence and aphasia followed the ictal period. The ictal EEG recording taken while eating is in *Figure 5* and a spontaneous seizure recorded during sleep is showed in *Figure 6*. Her high-resolution MRI study was normal (*Figure 7*).

Their 24-year-old aunt has been having only partial seizures induced by eating since 17 years of age. Since then she has presented about 10 episodes, most of them occurring at lunchtime. They are characterized by staring, oroalimentary automatisms and loss of consciousness for 30 seconds. Her interictal EEG and MRI were unremarkable. Carbamazepine (400 mg/day) led to seizure control for three years. In her second

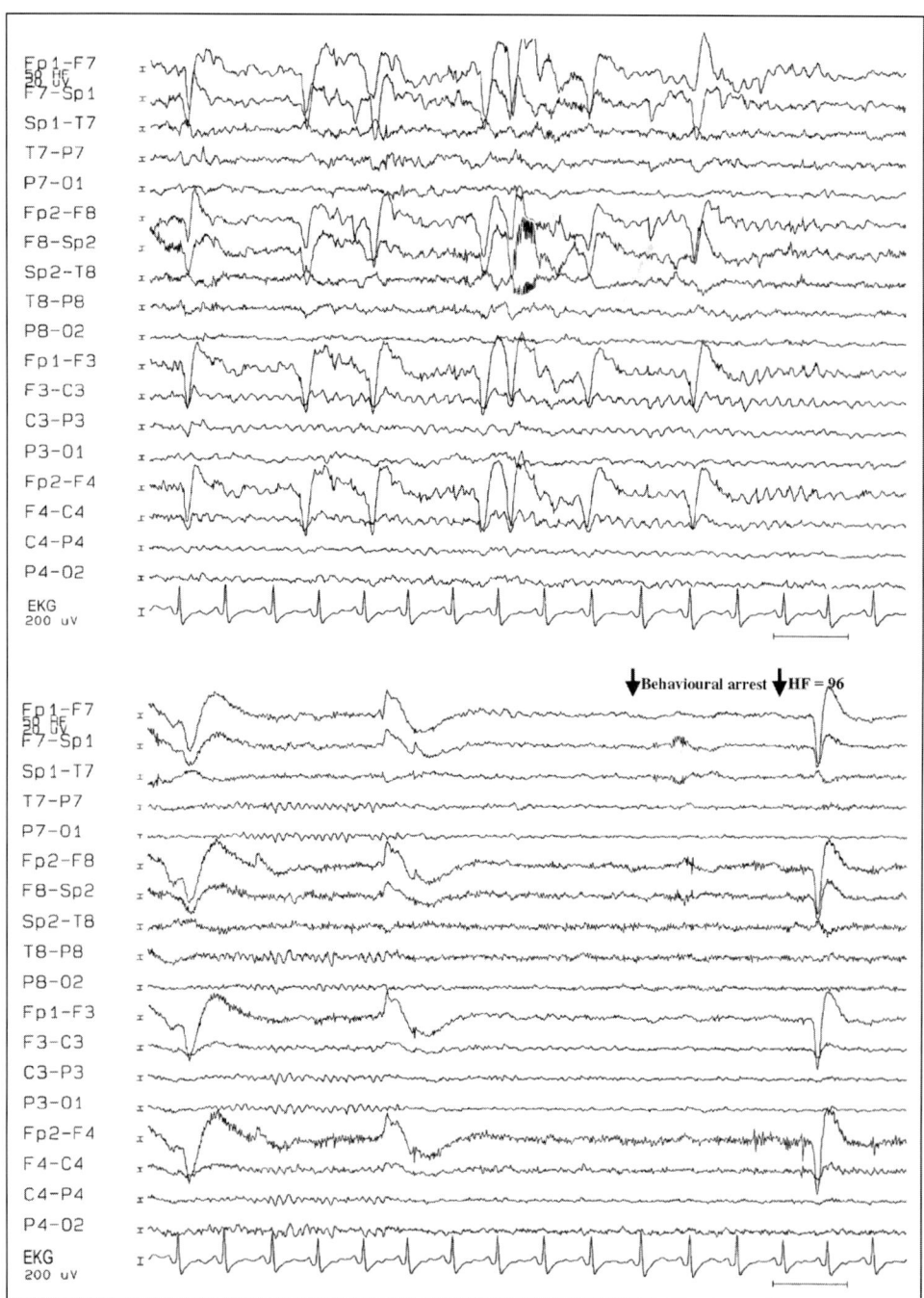

Figure 1a. Ictal EEG during seizure associated with eating. Since the beginning of the meal long runs of intermittent theta activity were recorded bilaterally, mainly over the anterior areas.

Figure 1b. About 7 minutes after the onset of the meal a low-voltage EEG substituted the theta runs till the end of a 90 s complex partial seizure.

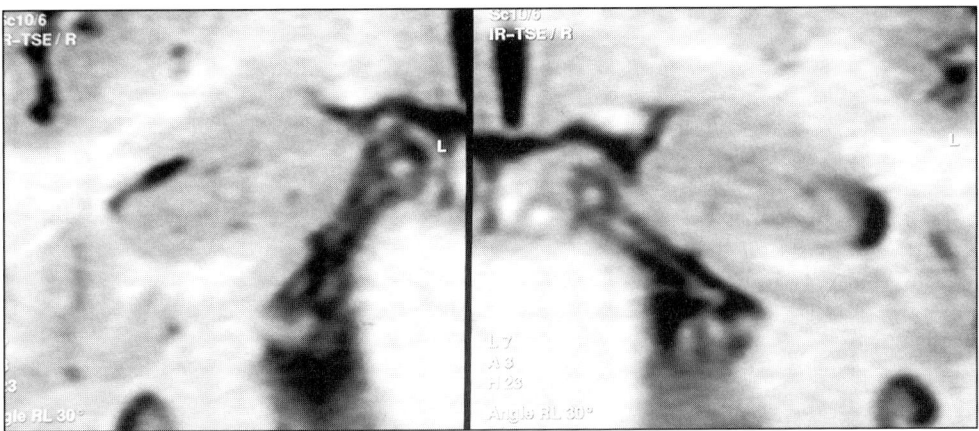

Figure 2. An inversion recovery MRI showing normal medial temporal structures.

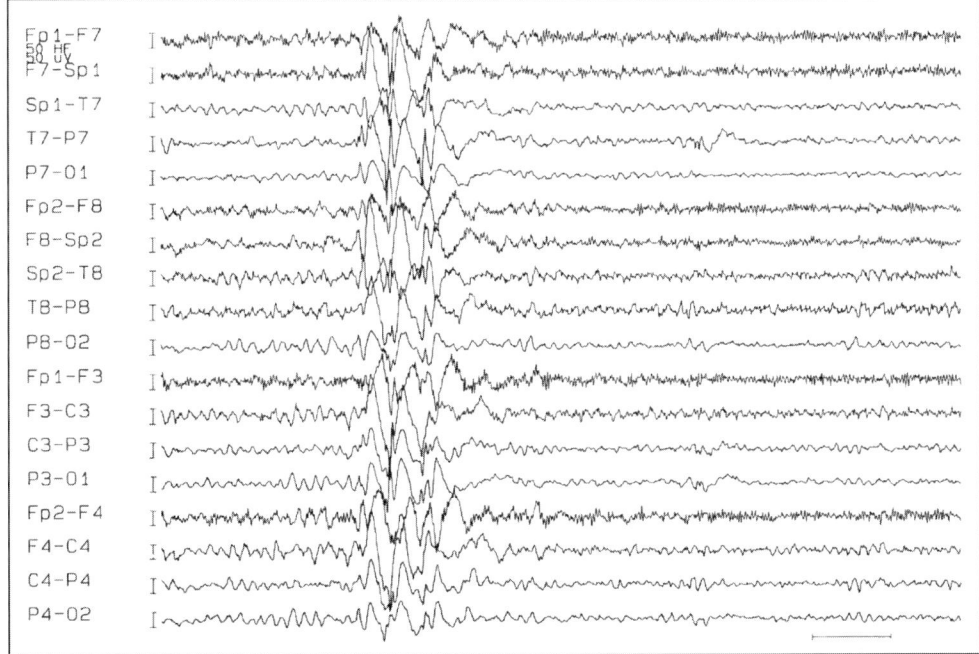

Figure 3. Generalised burst of spike-wave complexes recorded during wakefulness.

pregnancy, 1.2 years ago, barbexaclone 100 mg substituted carbamazepine. Her last complex partial seizure occurred two months ago, also at lunchtime but due to missing her medicine twice.

The pedigree and history of the other family members is summarised in *Figure 8*. Cases 3, 7 and 8 had seizures related to eating. Two men (cases 2 and 6) presented temporal lobe epilepsy and myoclonic juvenile epilepsy, respectively. Cases 1, 4 and 5 presented epilepsy whose seizures could not be classified.

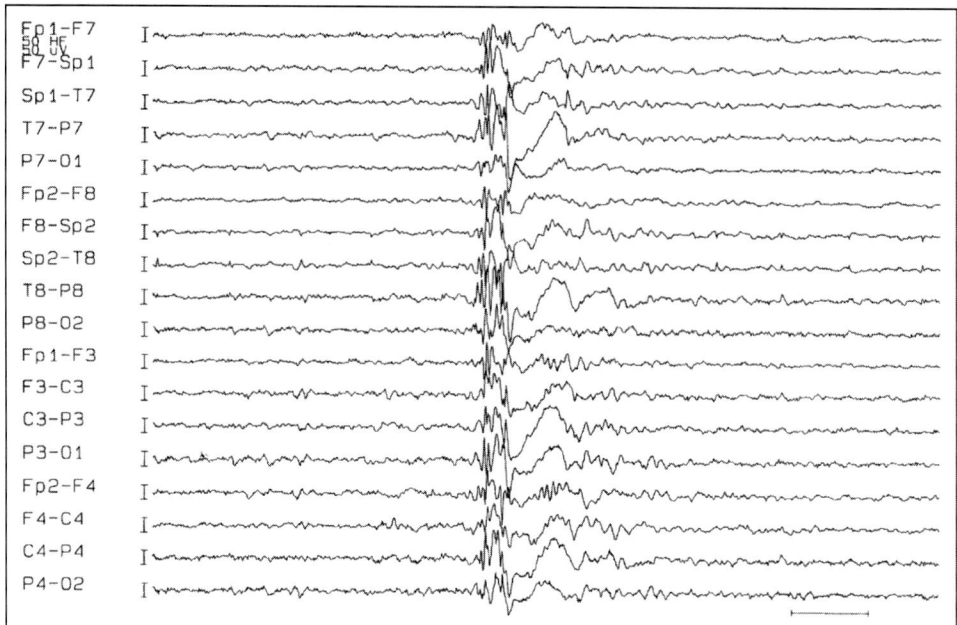

Figure 4. Generalised polyspike discharge recorded during sleep.

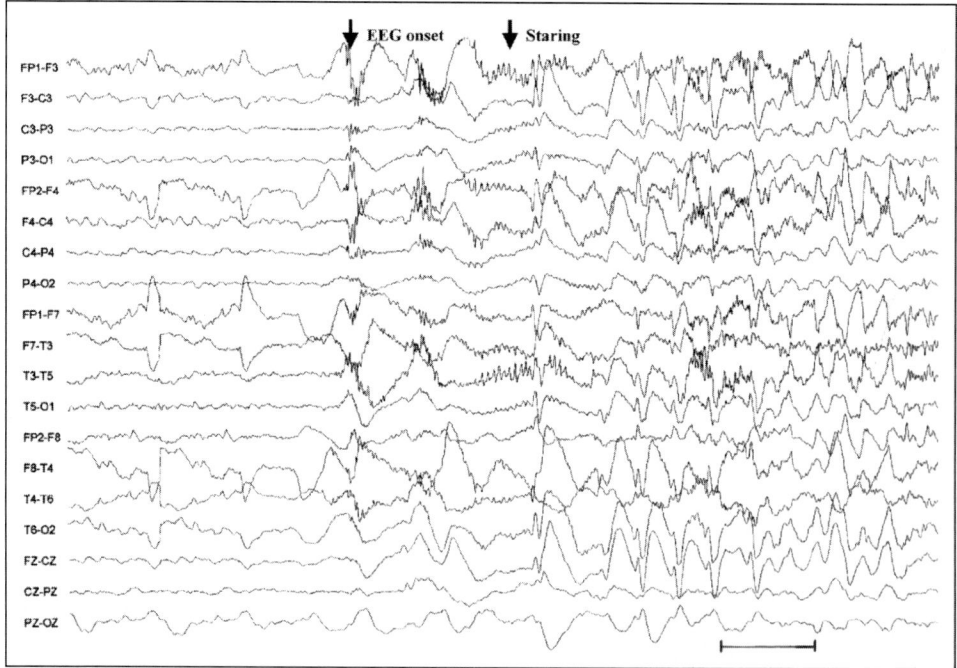

Figure 5. Ictal EEG during seizure associated with eating. Generalised spike, sharp and slow wave complexes followed a 3 s initial desynchronization of the EEG with low-voltage fast-frequencies. Delta waves over the left hemisphere were recorded for several minutes during the postictal period.

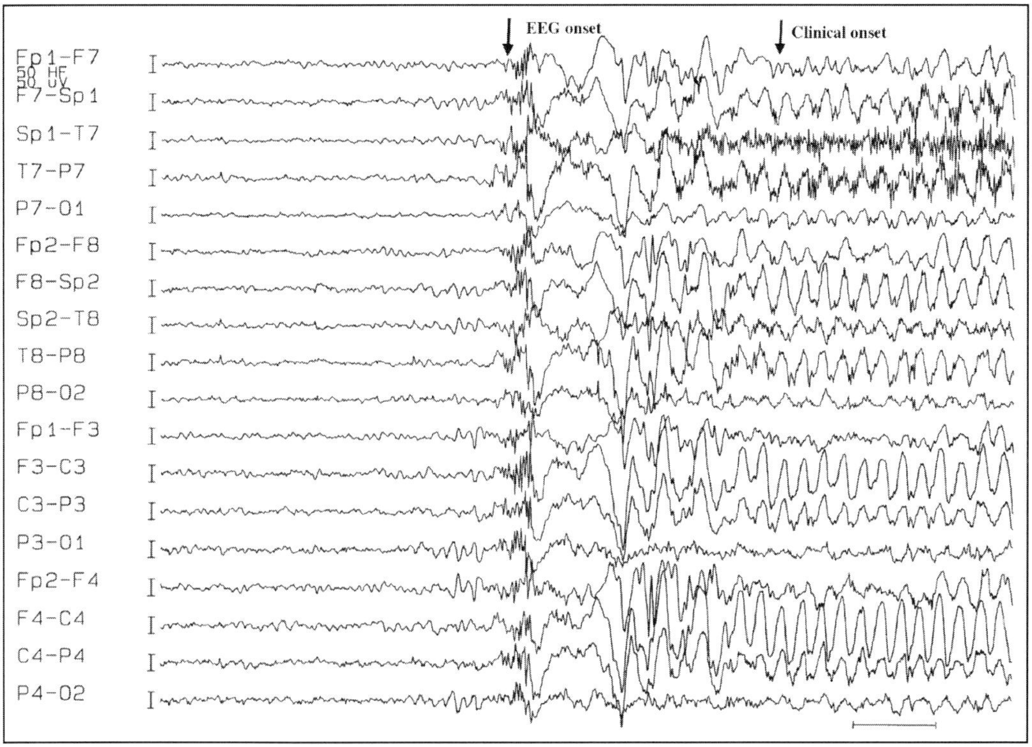

Figure 6. Ictal EEG during a spontaneous seizure recorded during sleep. Notice the similarity of the ictal pattern with the eating-induced seizure.

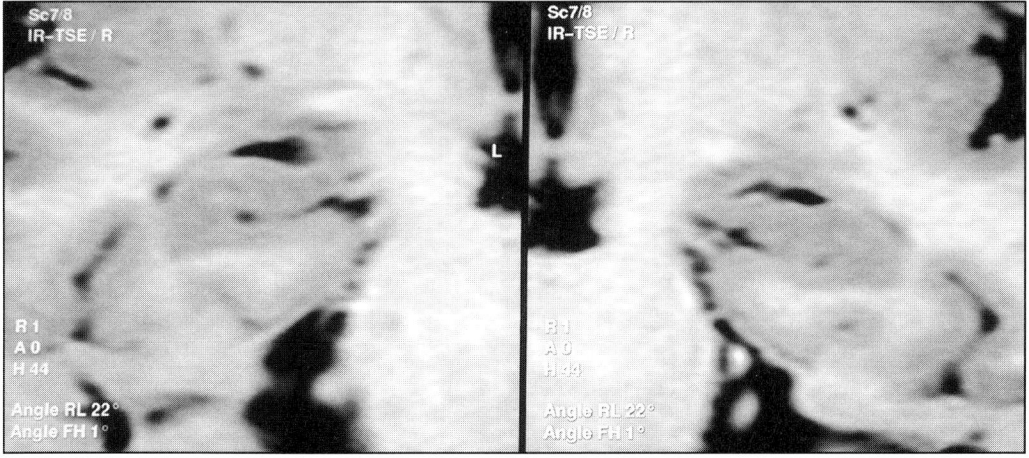

Figure 7. MRI emphasizing the medial temporal lobe structures did not show any abnormality.

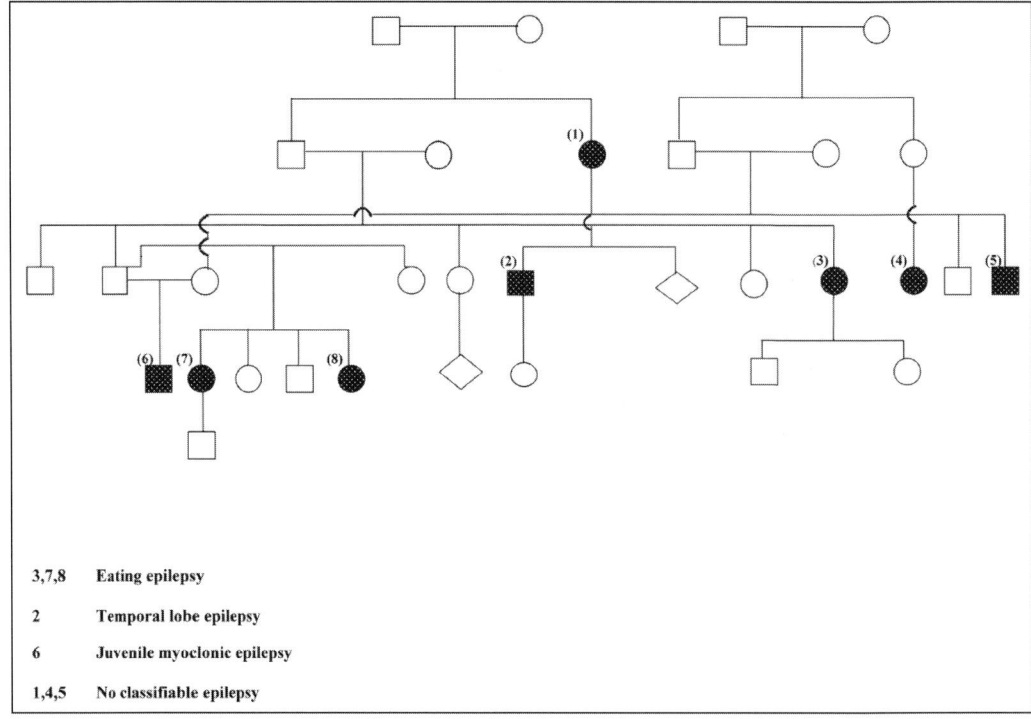

Figure 8. Pedigree of the patients with eating epilepsy (cases 3, 7 and 8) whose histories are given in the text. Histories of the other individuals with epilepsy in this family: (2) A 47-year-old man presented seizure onset at 12. Blurring vision, loss of consciousness and falling with rapid return characterized the episodes. Initially occurring 3-4/day, there was some improvement with carbamazepine (1000 mg/day). At present the frequency is 1/week. The EEG showed sharp waves over the left temporal lobe and the MRI was normal. (6) A 24-year-old man, a half brother of cases 7 and 8, had presented myoclonic jerks and tonic-clonic seizures since the age of 15. Valproate (1000 mg/day) led to seizure control. On EEG bursts of diffuse irregular spike-wave complexes were recorded and the MRI was normal. (1), (4) and (5) are family members with epilepsy whose seizures could not be classified. Cases 4 and 5 are only blood related to case 6.

■ Discussion

Eating seizures have been reported as present mainly in temporal lobe epilepsy. Rémillard et al. (1989) proposed two clinical syndromes of eating seizures, differentiating temporolimbic from extralimbic, suprasylvian seizure onset. Temporolimbic seizures activated by eating are considered a complex reflex epilepsy, and therefore need elaborated triggering stimuli acting for a long latency in order to provoke a fit. Seizures induced by eating of suprasylvian origin are seen in patients with lesions of the somatosensory cortex and are triggered by proprioceptive or somatosensory afferences during eating resembling those described with simple reflex epilepsies. In this modality, eating less constantly activates the seizures.

Eating epilepsy with temporolimbic onset initiated in the second decade of life is more common in males and has been associated with a family history of epilepsy in 28%-50% of the cases (Nagaraja & Chand, 1984; Senanayake, 1990b). In most of the published series, family members of patients with eating epilepsy present seizures not related to eating (Nagaraja & Chand, 1984; Ahuja et al., 1988; Koul et al., 1989).

In the pioneer series of 20 cases of familial eating epilepsy, Senanayake (1990a) emphasized a remarkable degree of intra-family consistency with regard to age at onset, symptomatology of seizures and timing of eating seizures. The male/female ratio in his series was 13:7 and the median age at seizure onset was 17.

In this particular family all individuals with eating seizures were female and started having complex partial seizures with similar symptomatology mainly related to eating (yet at different mealtimes) in the second decade of life, although both focal and generalised discharges were recorded in interictal and ictal EEGs.

Previous reports have described both partial and generalised seizures being triggered by eating. Although most series described partial seizures originating in the temporal lobes, generalised seizures have also been reported (Aguglia & Tinuper, 1983; Cirignotta et al., 1977). The patient reported by Fiol et al. (1986) had both complex partial and generalised seizures. The same is seen in relation to interictal recording. Ahuja et al. (1988) reported temporal foci in four of their 17 patients and Nagaraja & Chand (1984) found a regional irritative zone involving the temporal lobes in seven out of 13 cases. The interictal EEG in 18 of the 20 patients with familial eating epilepsy reported by Senanayake (1990a) showed focal discharges in either or both temporal areas. Nevertheless, generalised interictal discharges have been reported in other nonfamilial cases (Ahuja et al., 1980; Reder & Wright, 1982).

Regarding possible pathogenesis of familial eating epilepsy, Senanayake (1990a), based on clinical and interictal EEG data, suggested that in his series the epilepsy was probably idiopathic in all individuals but one and recognized the genetic susceptibility of this partial form of epilepsy which would act in conjunction with environmental factors in triggering the seizures. Favouring this hypothesis, siblings of each of his nine families had been brought up together sharing the same food and having similar eating habits.

Environmental and ethnic factors have been considered as important in eating epilepsy. Chemburkar and Desai (1977) described seven patients whose reflex seizures occurred only when eating at home, and first mentioned the possibility that a familiar atmosphere of home could play an important part in seizure precipitation since none of their patients suffered any event while eating out of their homes. Ahuja et al. (1988) have also emphasized the importance of familiar environment in seizure precipitation when describing seven out of 17 cases whose seizures occurred exclusively when eating at home. Most of the published series came from India and Sri Lanka where both genetic and ethnic factors have been implied in the pathogenic mechanisms. Among them, bulky meals rich in carbohydrates have been postulated as possible triggering factors (Senanayake, 1990b).

In this family, of Portuguese ancestry, the aunt had never lived together with her nieces, a fact that favours the importance of genetic traits in the genesis of the epilepsy. On the other hand, individuals of the same siblings present different EEG patterns and epilepsy syndromes. Therefore, case 7 presents focal epileptiform discharges on EEG while her sister (case 8) presents mainly generalised epileptiform discharges in interictal and ictal EEG, while their half brother (case 6) presented a typical form of juvenile myoclonic epilepsy. Interestingly, co-existence of idiopathic generalised and focal epilepsies have been reported in reflex epilepsies. Radhakrishnan et al. (1995) diagnosed a co-occurrence with juvenile myoclonic epilepsy in four of their 20 patients with primary reading epilepsy and Mayer and Wolf (1997) observed it in an additional three cases. Nevertheless, seizure precipitation by both praxis and talking/reading in juvenile myoclonic epilepsy has also been reported by Wolf and Mayer (2000). These observations as to how focal the manifestations of generalised epilepsies can be raise the question of how generalised the focal semiology of the seizures described in this family with eating seizures came about. There is also a discussion as to how large the regional recruitment to reach a "critical mass" needs to be to produce the clinical signs in eating-induced seizures. The same is also the case of other forms of seizures precipitated by specific stimuli as in seizures induced by reading whose generation is neither focal nor "generalised" but related to a set of functionally interactive anatomical sites with a certain amount of clustering at the motor and language areas of the dominant hemisphere (Wolf, 2000).

A variety of afferent stimuli has been implied as triggering factors in eating seizures: simple presentation of food, somatosensory and proprioceptive inputs from hand movements, tasting, chewing, swallowing and gastric distension as well as affective and emotional stimuli. The complexity of such stimuli certainly suggests the activation of wide encephalic areas including the hypothalamic nuclei and brainstem structures involved in the cephalic phase of digestion (Robertson & Fariello, 1979; Reder & Wright, 1982; Rémillard et al., 1998). The seizures recorded in both sisters here described corroborated this complexity, since the simple presentation of food and/or proprioceptive afferences from hand and arm movements seem to have represented the main precipitating factor in the seizure documented during dinner in the first case, while in the second, gastric distension certainly could be considered at least one of the implied factors as her recorded seizure during lunch occurred only at the end of a prolonged heavy meal.

In relation to the etiology, previously considered acquired disorders, different forms of partial epilepsies have been reported in families. Among them, temporal lobe epilepsy has recently been the object of important studies (Berkovic et al., 1994; Cendes et al., 1998; Kobayashi et al., 2001). While Berkovic et al. (1994) described an idiopathic and benign form of familial temporal lobe epilepsy, Kobayashi et al. (2001) based on a large nonsurgical familial series of temporal lobe epilepsy described a spectrum of hippocampal abnormalities and clinical course of temporal lobe epilepsy, as there were individuals with few seizures to refractory epilepsy.

Since our patients do not present clinical signs of neurological dysfunction and any lesion on MRI, despite the difficulty in seizure control and the high seizure frequency observed in two of them, their eating temporolimbic seizures may represent a manifestation of an idiopathic form of temporal lobe epilepsy. In these cases, the temporolimbic structures might be seen as a receptive region for the afferences involved in reflex eating seizures as the occipital cortex is involved in photosensitivity of the generalised epilepsies and the associative areas of the temporoparietal lobes are involved in complex reflex epilepsies. In this family we believe that we are not confronted with an eating epilepsy syndrome, but with a strong genetic trait that gives susceptibility to eating seizures. However, the degree of this genetic trait determining the seizure threshold varied among the three affected members of this family. Notwithstanding the remarkable similarity in seizure onset and symptoms, although with different degrees of epilepsy severity, clinical heterogeneity was also seen in these cases since there were members of the same family with eating seizures besides temporal lobe epilepsy not related to eating and juvenile myoclonic epilepsy.

Acknowledgements

This paper received a grant from FAPESP (Fundação de Amparo à Pesquisa do Estado de São Paulo), São Paulo, Brazil. The authors thank the Directory of the Hospital Alemão Oswaldo Cruz, São Paulo, for their support.

References

1. Aguglia U, Tinuper P. Eating seizures. *Eur Neurol* 1983; 22: 227-31.
2. Ahuja GK, Mohandas S, Narayanaswamy AS. Eating epilepsy. *Epilepsia* 1980; 21: 85-9.
3. Ahuja GK, Pauranik A, Behari M, Prasad K. Eating epilepsy. *J Neurol* 1988; 235: 444-7.
4. Berkovic SF, Howell RA, Hopper JL. Familial temporal lobe epilepsy: a new syndrome with adolescent/adult onset and a benign course. In: Wolf P, ed. *Epileptic seizures and syndromes*. London: John Libbey, 1994; 257-63.
5. Cendes F, Lopes-Cendes I, Andermann E, Andermann F. Familial temporal lobe epilepsy: a clinically heterogeneous syndrome. *Neurology* 1998; 50: 554-7.
6. Chemburkar JA, Desai A. Reflex epilepsy. *Bull Jaslok Hosp Res Unit*, Bombay, India 1977; 1: 197-200.
7. Cirignotta F, Marcacci G, Lugaresi E. Epileptic seizures precipitated by eating. *Epilepsia* 1977; 18: 445-9.
8. Fiol ME, Leppik IE, Pretzel K. Eating epilepsy: EEG and clinical study. *Epilepsia* 1986; 27: 441-5.
9. Kobayashi E, Lopes-Cendes I, Guerreiro CAM, Sousa SC, Guerreiro MM, Cendes F. Seizure outcome and hippocampal atrophy in familial mesial temporal lobe epilepsy. *Neurology* 2001; 56: 166-72.
10. Koul R, Koul S, Razdan S. Eating epilepsy. *Acta Neurol Scand* 1989; 80: 78-80.
11. Mayer T, Wolf P. Reading epilepsy: related to juvenile myoclonic epilepsy? *Epilepsia* 1997; 38 (suppl. 3): 18-9.
12. Nagaraja D, Chand RP. Eating epilepsy. *Clin Neurol Neurosurg* 1984; 86: 95-9.
13. Radhakrishnan K, Silbert PL, Klass DW. Reading epilepsy. An appraisal of 20 patients diagnosed at the Mayo Clinic, Rochester, Minnesota, between 1949 and 1989, and delineation of the epileptic syndrome. *Brain* 1995; 118: 75-89.

14. Reder AT, Wright FS. Epilepsy evoked by eating: the role of peripheral input. *Neurology* 1982; 32: 1065-9.
15. Rémillard GM, Andermann F, Zifkin BG, Olivier A, Rasmussen T. Eating epilepsy: a study of ten surgically treated patients suggests the presence of two separate syndromes. In: Beaumanoir A, Gastaut H, Naquet R, eds. *Reflex seizures and reflex epilepsies*. Geneva: Médecine et Hygiène, 1989; 289-300.
16. Rémillard GM, Zifkin BG, Andermann F. Seizures induced by eating. In: Zifkin BG, Andermann F, Beaumanoir A, Rowan J, eds. *Reflex epilepsies and reflex seizures*. Philadelphia: Lippincott-Raven, 1998; 227-40.
17. Robertson WC, Fariello RG. Eating epilepsy associated with a deep forebrain glioma. *Ann Neurol* 1979; 6: 271-3.
18. Senanayake N. Familial eating epilepsy. *J Neurol* 1990a; 237: 388-91.
19. Senanayake N. "Eating epilepsy" – a reappraisal. *Epilepsy Res* 1990b; 5: 74-9.
20. Wolf P. Activation of seizures by reading and praxis. In: Lüders HO, Noachtar S, eds. *Epileptic seizures. Pathophysiology and clinical semiology*. Philadelphia: Churchill Livingstone, 2000; 609-14.
21. Wolf P, Mayer T. Juvenile myoclonic epilepsy: a syndrome challenging syndromic concepts? In: Schmitz B, Sander T, eds. *Juvenile myoclonic epilepsy. The Janz syndrome*. Petersfield: Wrightson, 2000; 33-9.
22. Zifkin BG, Andermann F, Rémillard GM. Epilepsy with seizures induced by eating. In: Wolf P, ed. *Epileptic seizures and syndromes*. London: John Libbey, 1994; 99-105.

Motor reflex epilepsy induced by touch and movement

A. Biraben, E. Doury, J.M. Scarabin

Service de Neurologie, CHU Pontchaillou, Rennes

■ Definition

Epileptic seizures may be induced by a combination of events often recognized or suspected by the patient or physician. Metabolic disorders, variations in hormone levels, drug intake, or more subtle factors (*e.g.* psychic perturbations, emotions) may be involved. For most patients, the multiplicity and complexity of these events makes it impossible to predict seizures. At best "favourable" conditions can be described.

For certain patients, however, epileptic phenomena are induced by identified stimuli. Such patients have reflex epilepsy, which can be triggered by one or more stimulating events. If the seizures are induced uniquely by such stimuli, the patient is said to have pure reflex epilepsy. If the seizures are induced by the recognized stimuli but also occur spontaneously, the patient is said to have epilepsy with reflex seizures.

In patients with perirolandic reflex epilepsy, seizures are induced by a variety of events: touching the skin a certain way, specific movements, food intake, brushing teeth, cognitive activities, etc. [1].

Different types of seizures can be induced: partial motor or sensorial seizures, generalised seizures, monoclonal seizures. Such seizures may also be observed in patients with epilepsia partialis continua [2].

■ Seizures induced by touch or movement

Among the 800 epilepsy patients treated in our centre since 1992, only eight (1%) presented reflex epilepsy induced by touch or movement (not including startle epilepsy). The first three case reports presented here have been described in detail in an earlier publication [3].

■ Case Reports

Patient #1

This 20-year-old man had experienced epileptic seizures since the age of seven years. Seizures occurred daily and were the same since the beginning. They were generally triggered by the patient himself. A refractory period of several hours after each seizure prevented a subsequent seizure, otherwise triggered by contact with clothes. The reflex zone was located in the lower part of the chest on the left side. Tapping this zone regularly triggered the seizure which started by localised tingling that spread progressively and rapidly. The sensation extended to the entire chest, then to the left arm, followed by tonic contraction of the left hemithorax, the left arm, and finally the right half of the body. The seizure terminated with a few clonic movements of the proximal portion of the left arm. The patient remained conscious throughout the seizure.

Sensory evoked potentials (SEP) remained normal when the reflex zone was stimulated. Brain magnetic resonance imaging (MRI) was normal as was the interictal EEG. The ictal EEG demonstrated low-voltage polymorphic rhythmic spikes in the central region and in the vertex during the tonic phase. This patient underwent stereoelectroencephalography (SEEG) using the method described by Bancaud and Talairach [4]. When the reflex zone was stimulated, the deep electrodes recorded slow waves on which were superimposed rapid discharges in the parietal sensory cortex and the rolandic motor cortex in phase with the tapping on the chest wall. A rapid discharge then appeared in the right sensorimotor cortex and the left motor cortex during the tonic contraction *(for details see ref. 3)*.

The patient was given topiramate in 1993 and since that time has experienced only one seizure. He has been able to continue his college education and has not undergone surgery.

Patient #2

This 18-year-old woman had epileptic seizures since the age of 15 years. Her family history was uneventful. Her seizures were almost identical since the beginning, with exceptional secondary generalisations. The physical exam was normal. The reflex zone, located in the left iliac fossa, was activated by contact with clothes when walking or by massage.

Spontaneously, or after stimulation, the patient developed paresthesia described as a heavy feeling in the reflex zone that extended to the entire lower limb. Tonic contraction then started in the left foot and progressively spread to the abdominal muscles, sometimes reaching the thorax and the left shoulder leading to abduction of the shoulder. The patient remained conscious and memory was not perturbed. She was able to talk during seizures. After seizures she presented a sensorial deficit in the left lower limb. Spontaneous seizures were frequent. Self-sustained seizures occasionally led to secondary status epilepticus.

SEP recordings were normal, even during stimulation of the reflex zone. The brain MRI was normal and a recent FLAIR sequence MRI with 3-D reconstruction was also normal. The interictal EEG was normal and the ictal tracing showed rapid spikes located in the central and right parasagittal areas.

Recently, the seizures have occurred in clusters; medication (topiramate and lamotrigine) has enabled seizure-free periods of several months. This patient was able to continue schooling and is currently working as an assistant for elderly persons.

Patient #3

This 24-year-old man had experienced epileptic seizures since the age of 13 years. His personal history included a benign head trauma.

Seizures lasting 20 to 30 seconds occurred four or five times a day, more often when sleeping, and had been the same from the beginning. During the day, seizures were triggered by flexion-extension movements and large-amplitude rotation of the left shoulder. The physical exam was normal. The seizures began by a sensation of electricity running along the medial and posterior aspect of the left arm. The patient then lost sensitivity in the rest of the arm and finally became unable to control his left arm. These events were sometimes followed by propagation of the electrical sensation to the anterior aspect of the left chest and the left thigh, and subsequent loss of sensitivity in these regions and tonic contraction of the left arm and incapacity to speak. The seizures terminated by clonic shaking of the left arm. Consciousness was not perturbed and secondary generalised seizures were rare. The patient could trigger seizures voluntarily.

SEP and brain MRI were normal. The interictal EEG showed low-voltage polymorphic spikes in the right central region. No complementary invasive exploration has been attempted to date.

Patient #4

This 41-year-old man experienced his first seizures at the age of nine years. He was given Phenobarbital and remained seizure-free to the age of 18 years. Seizures, which occurred several times a day, were sometimes triggered by active or passive movements of the toes or the left foot; other seizures were probably spontaneous. The neurological exam was normal. Seizures began by a flush of the left leg followed by an ascending sensation to the back and arm. The patient's left leg then began to move and his head turned to the right. The patient remained conscious but fell if he could not grasp a support. He had transient paralysis of the left leg during the postictal period.

The interictal EEG was normal. The ictal EEG showed a bilateral discharge starting by right frontal spikes which were visible despite artefacts. The SEP recordings showed a retarded early response and giant late responses favouring, in our opinion, a lesion associated with hyperexcitability. The FLAIR sequence MRI showed a high intensity signal deep in the central gyrus highly suggestive of a small area of Taylor dysplasia (*Figure 1*). The patient has preferred to abstain from any further investigations due to the risk of paralysis if surgery were attempted.

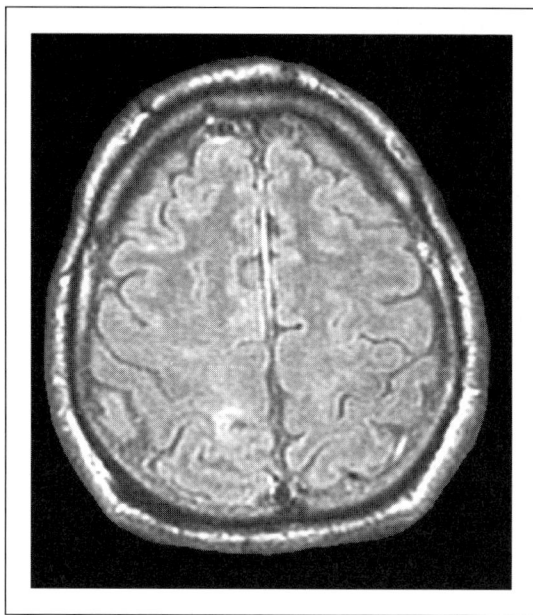

Figure 1. Patient FH.
MRI FLAIR sequence showing the abnormal signal in the lower limb motor region.

■ Synopsis of clinical presentations

Touch-induced seizures

The epileptic seizure is triggered when a limited area of skin, which in our experience remains unchanged over time, is touched in a particular manner. As illustrated in our case reports, the sensitivity of the trigger zone may vary, stimulation inducing seizures more or less readily. Some patients have a refractory period after the seizure, while others exhibit an unexplained variability in sensitivity. Different body areas may be involved.

In some patients, the trigger zone has to be stimulated repeatedly to induce a seizure, suggesting that a temporal summation might be involved. For others, the seizure occurs suddenly or unexpectedly, in which case somesthetic phenomena are not observed before seizure onset.

The trigger zones are sensitive to different types of stimulation, *e.g.* tapping, rubbing, massage. A particular rhythm, well recognized by the patient, may be particularly effective in inducing the seizure. For some patients a seizure always occurs if the trigger zone is touched at this rhythm, irrespective of the type of stimulation. Spontaneous formication or a heavy feeling are also reported in the trigger zone, independently of seizures.

Movement-induced seizures

It is not clear whether touch-induced and movement-induced seizures are different phenomena or two presentations of a unique phenomenon. Movement-induced seizures always involve the same joint or group of joints in a given patient. Different types of movements can induce seizures: simple movements, complex or ample movements, sometimes passive movements, and, exceptionally, even ideation of movement. A specific rhythm or a sudden movement after a rest period may be required to trigger the seizure. In all published cases, small lesions in the region of the rolandic and pre-rolandic cortex (supplementary motor area) [5, 9] were found. At that time no lesion was seen on MRI, but ictal EEG showed abnormal discharge localised in the central region.

Seizures induced by both touch and movement

When seizures can be induced by either touch or movement in a given patient, the clinical presentation of the induced seizures is quite similar. Whether spontaneous or provoked, the seizures are short lived. The trigger zone and the region implicated in the triggering movement are very close or the same.

Types of seizures

Few case reports concern reflex seizures induced by touch or movement [5-9]. The seizures are typically brief, lasting 20 to 30 seconds. Lishman et al. [8] noted that seizure precipitation could be related to the context in which the movement occurred. In some patients sudden movement or movements after a period of rest appeared more likely to precipitate seizures. Conversely, preparation for movement and the slow initiation of action tended to reduce seizure or abort seizures. Falconer et al. [5] reported a patient who could defer seizure by voluntary relaxation of the quadriceps muscle; in this patient a complete resolution of symptoms was obtained by surgical resection of a meningocerebral cicatrix anterior to the precentral gyrus. Wolf and Dockweiler [6] described deconditioning therapy in a patient with tonic versive seizures precipitated by touch. Kochen [7] reported reflex seizures beginning with localised myoclonus. Atonic manifestations have also been reported in two patients [11] with tonic and generalised seizures. In both cases ictal EEG showed bilateral polyspikes. These clinical and EEG manifestations differed from our observations and indicate widespread brain lesions. They do not correspond to the pure epilepsies originating in the sensorimotor cortex and triggered by movements.

The dysaesthesia the patients describe in the trigger zone may be a seizure equivalent or a sign of a functional disorder subsequent to activity in the brain lesion. The clinical signs of these reflex seizures vary from simple myoclonus to motor and/or sensorial seizures exhibiting jacksonian propagation, a sign of the essential involvement of the primary sensorimotor cortex. The motor symptoms predominate in the proximal portion of the limbs initially. Clonic movements often occur thereafter. Secondary generalisation does occur, but exceptionally. Some patients have a refractory period. In others seizure-induced movement during a period of hyperexcitability appears to be sufficient to trigger the next movement-induced seizure. The first seizure might also function like a primer, setting off a cortical pacemaker which sustains regularly repeated seizures. In the first case, each seizure is triggered by the preceding seizure while in the second case the seizures (often myoclonus) occur regularly from the start, the preceding seizure having little or no influence.

■ Pathophysiology

The distinction between touch-induced and movement-induced seizures would appear to be rather artificial since, as illustrated in our case reports, certain patients experience identical seizures triggered by either type of stimuli. A certain number of elements – sensorimotor symptoms, jacksonian propagation, localisation of the EEG anomalies – converge towards an implication of the motor regions in both touch-induced and movement-induced seizures [5-8]. The motor regions involved are the rolandic or primary sensorimotor cortex, or closely related regions such as the supplementary motor area as described in certain cases with identified lesions [5, 10].

The specific anatomic and functional features of the involved region(s) probably explain seizure onset. In these regions, the anatomic structures and physiological functions involved in receptive and motor effector activities are closely interrelated. More distant, and thus slower, regulatory influences can be shunted via direct rapid interconnections.

Somesthetic afferents transmitting external stimuli directly from the skin or joints reach the motor processing centres where their final target always are effector neurons in area 4 [12, 13]. If their activation threshold is abnormally low, these different influences can trigger epileptic seizures. This mechanism would explain not only seizures related directly to somatognosis, but also seizures triggered by preparing for a movement or actually performing the movement.

Different mechanisms could be involved:

- Rolandic hyperexcitability, probably related to a local cortical anomaly. Several cases of reflex epilepsy with lesions situated in the rolandic and motor region (including the supplementary motor area) have been reported [14, 15]. Very small areas of focal dysplasia could be expected in these cryptogenic cases where classical imaging would be "normal" because the foci are too small to be visualized with current techniques, but with an identifiable electrophysiological expression on in-situ recordings. This was the case in our first patient where surface SEP tracings were normal but showed polymorphic spikes on the recordings of the deep cortex situated in the central gyrus when the cutaneous trigger zone was stimulated.

- Primary implication of the sensory cortex. Dysfunction of the sensory cortex would explain why stimulating the skin produces an abnormal sensation in these patients who also often report signs of sensorial disorders at the beginning of their seizures. The presence of abnormal giant potentials on the EEG and SEEG is another argument favouring hyperexcitability of the primary sensory cortex. As in our fourth patient, these giant evoked potentials are actually the second P1-N2 part of the somesthetic response, the first part being normal. They could reflect an intracortical phenomenon such as discharge of pyramidal cells as suggested by

Shibazki [16] or cells which are not primary effector cells but directly connected to them [17]. The hypothesis of a hyperactive transcortical reflex loop has also been mentioned, particularly in certain cases of myoclonic epilepsy [18]. Definite confirmation has not been obtained, but this suspected mechanism could explain certain cases of reflex epilepsy manifested by sensory symptoms rather than seizures. For certain authors, giant evoked potentials and premyoclonic potentials recorded in epilepsia partialis continua would follow the same circuit. In a recent publication devoted to the physiology of reflex myoclonia, patients with progressive myoclonic epilepsy exhibited this abnormal reactivity of the sensorimotor cortex in response to magnetic stimulation. Normal SEP latency was associated with late giant spikes and decreased physiological inhibition [19].

- The role of subcortical structures most likely implicated in these seizures remains unknown. These structures might play a facilitating role via dysfunction of the inhibitory systems, even if the focalisation of the clinical signs is not in favour of this mechanism. A certain degree of somatotopic representation is known to exist in these structures.

Seizures induced by movement differ from startle epilepsy in several ways, as already proposed by Vignal *et al.* [3]. In movement-induced seizures no startle is seen; in startle epilepsy extensive damage of frontoparietal cortex are responsible for the seizures. Conversely, small lesions are found in movement-induced seizures or the cause remains unknown (may be linked to focal cortical dysplasia). On the other hand, perinatal encephalopathy represents the main etiological factor in startle epilepsy; at least, clinical seizures pattern are different: they are initially less sudden, in seizures induced by movement, and the motor signs are often preceded by localised sensory manifestation with a jacksonian march. On the other hand the clinical manifestations of the attacks in paroxysmal kinesigenic choreoathetosis (PKC) cannot be taken as a definitive argument against their possible epileptic nature, even more so because localised dysesthetic manifestations have also been reported. The nature of these manifestations does not seem to be epileptic; no EEG abnormalities have been reported interictally or even at the time of the attacks.

■ Conclusion

The characteristic features of touch-induced and movement-induced epilepsy are very similar. The normal sensory evoked potentials recorded in certain patients could be explained by the deep localisation of the abnormal generator (deep in gyri). A certain number of questions remain open concerning the pathophysiological mechanisms of these seizures. Is the initial element hyperexcitation, leading to afferent overflow which is not inhibited because the subcortical system is deficient? Does the hyperexcitability involve the sensory cortex or the motor cortex? Is there a circuit between the sensory and motor cortex that might allow the development of self-sustaining seizures?

We therefore believe reflex sensorimotor seizures to constitute an entity different from both PKC and startle epilepsy.

References

1. Wieser HG. Seizure induction in reflex seizures and reflex epilepsy. In: Zifkin BG, Andermann F, Beaumanoir A, Rowan AJ, eds. *Reflex epilepsies and reflex seizures. Adv Neurol Vol. 75.* Philadelphia: Lippincott-Raven, 1998; 69-85.
2. Biraben A, Chauvel P. Epilepsia partialis continua. In: Engel J Jr, Pedley TA, eds. *Epilepsy: a comprehensive textbook.* Philadelphia: Lippincott-Raven, 1997; 2447-53.
3. Vignal JP, Biraben A, Chauvel P, Reutens D. Reflex partial seizures of sensoriotor cortex (including cortical reflex myoclonus and startle epilepsy). In: Zifkin BG, Andermann F, Beaumanoir A, Rowan AJ, eds. *Reflex epilepsies and reflex seizures. Adv Neurol Vol. 75.* Philadelphia: Lippincott-Raven, 1998; 207-26.
4. Bancaud J, Angelergues R, Bernouilli C, Bonis A, Bordas-Ferrer M, Bresson M, Buser P, Covello L, Morel P, Szikla G, Takeda A, Talairach J. Functional stereotaxic exploration (SEEG) of epilepsy. *Electroencephalogr Clin Neurophysiol* 1970; 28: 85-6.
5. Falconer MA, Driver MV, Serafetinides EA. Seizures induced by movement: report of case relieved by operation. *J Neurol Neurosurg Psychiatr* 1963; 26: 300-7.
6. Wolf P, Dockweiler U. Deconditioning therapy in a patient with versive seizures precipitated by touch. In: Beaumanoir A, Gastaut H, Naquet R, eds. *Reflex seizures and reflex epilepsies.* Geneva: Editions Médecine et Hygiène, 1989; 447-51.
7. Kochen S. Reflex epilepsy induced by movement, a case report. In: Beaumanoir A, Gastaut H, Naquet R, eds. *Reflex seizures and reflex epilepsies.* Geneva: Editions Médecine et Hygiène, 1989; 115-7.
8. Lishman WA, Symonds CP, Whitty GWM, Willison RG. Seizures induced by movement. *Brain* 1962; 85: 93-108.
9. Whitty CWM, Lishman WA, Fitzgibbon JP. Seizures induced by movement: a form of reflex epilepsy. *Lancet* 1964; 1: 1043-5.
10. Kennedy WA. Clinical and electroencephalographic aspects of epileptogenic lesions of the medial surface and superior border of cerebral hemisphere. *Brain* 1959; 85: 147-61.
11. Oller-Daurella L, Oller Ferrer-Vidal L. Seizures induced by voluntary movements. In: Beaumanoir A, Gastaut H, Naquet R, eds. *Reflex seizures and reflex epilepsies.* Geneva: Editions Médecine et Hygiène, 1959; 139-46.
12. Asanuma H, Rosen I. Topographical organization of the cortical efferent zones projecting to distal forelimb muscles in monkey Exp. *Brain Res* 1972; 14: 243-56.
13. Rosen I, Asanuma H. Peripheral afferent inputs to the forelimb area of the monkey motor cortex. *Exp Brain Res* 1972; 14: 257-73.
14. Penfield W, Erickson TC. *Epilepsy and cerebral localization.* Springfield, IL: CC Thomas, 1941; 27-8.
15. Forster FM, Penfield W, Jasper H, Madow L. Focal epilepsy, sensory precipitation and evoked cortical potentials. *Electroenceph Clin Neurophysiol* 1949; 1: 349-56.
16. Shibazaki H, Yamashita Y, Neshige R, Tobimatsu S, Fukui R. Pathogenesis of giant somatosensory evoked potential in progressive myoclonic epilepsy. *Brain* 1985; 108: 225-40.
17. Marsden CD. The physiology of myoclonus and its relation to epilepsy. *Res Clin Forum* 1980; 2: 31-46.
18. Shibazaki H, Yamashita Y, Kuroiwa Y. Electroencephalographic studies of myoclonus: myoclonus-related cortical spikes and high amplitude somatosensory evoked potentials. *Brain* 1978; 101: 447-60.
19. Manganotti P, Tamburin S, Zanette G, Fiaschi A. Hyperexcitable cortical responses in progressive myoclonic epilepsy a TMS study. *Neurology* 2001; 57: 1793-9.

Malformations of cortical development as a cause of reflex seizures: neurobiological insights

A. Palmini, P. Halasz*, I. Schaeffer**, Y. Takahashi***, A. Perez Jimenez****, F. Dubeau#, F. Andermann#, F. Rosenow*****, B. Fritsch*****

From the Porto Alegre Epilepsy Surgery Program, Hospital São Lucas, Pontificia Universidade Católica do Rio Grande do Sul (PUCRS), Porto Alegre, Brazil;
* National Institute of Psychiatry and Neurology, Budapest, Hungary
** Austin and Repatriation Medical Center, University of Melbourne, Australia;
*** Department of Pediatrics, Gifu Prefectural Hospital, Gifu, Japan;
**** Department of Pediatrics, Hospital del Niño Jesus, Madrid, Spain;
 # Department of Neurology and Neurosurgery, Montreal Neurological Institute and Hospital, McGill University, Montreal, Canada;
***** The Interdisciplinary Epilepsy Center, Department of Neurology, Philipps-University Marburg, Germany

Introduction

Malformations of cortical development (MCD) are often associated with medically refractory seizures in patients with focal or generalised epilepsies [1, 2]. From a group of disorders only rarely seen in clinical practice until the late '80s, MCD became an important entity in epileptology over the last decade, *pari passu* with advances in magnetic resonance imaging (MRI), which has allowed their identification *in vivo*. It became progressively clear that MCD represent a major aetiology of epilepsy, associated or not with cognitive or motor abnormalities, and it is likely that these entities are the underlying etiology of 15%-20% of epilepsies considered for surgical treatment in tertiary epilepsy centers [2, 3].

Some forms of MCD may be exceedingly epileptogenic, and are not only associated with medically refractory seizures, but also with a high prevalence of epilepsia partialis continua (EPC) and a frequent occurrence of continuous, rhythmic, or bursting epileptiform discharges in the electrographic recordings of these patients [1, 4-7]. These clinical findings have set the stage for the investigation of the pathogenetic mechanisms related to the epileptogenicity of MCD. Evidence that within these lesions there is an imbalance characterized by increased excitation and decreased inhibition has been accumulating in recent years, and scientific-based views of why MCD often lead to difficult-to-treat epilepsies are emerging. Several laboratories are independently demonstrating decreased numbers and deranged function of local circuit, inhibitory, intracortical interneurons, and also an excessive number of excitatory amino acid receptors [8-11]. The net result of these abnormalities would result in significant hyperexcitability.

There are different types of MCD, with variable pathogenesis, morphological features, and degree of epileptogenicity [1, 12, 13]. The common denominator is a developmental abnormality of the cortical mantle, which may be localised or more extensive over one or both hemispheres. These entities are caused by a variety of genetic or acquired disorders interfering at different points during embryogenesis. It is likely that type, timing, and degree of severity of interference during embryogenesis modulate the links between MCD and epilepsy.

Interestingly, one aspect that has not been formally studied is the potential of MCD to give rise to reflex seizures. The latter usually result from epileptogenic cortical tissue with a propensity to respond with abnormally increased electrical volleys to afferent stimuli, thus establishing hyperexcitable sensorimotor loops [14-16]. Because significant cortical hyperexcitability is a frequent feature of MCD, it would be a reasonable expectation that reflex seizures should occur with an increased frequency in patients harboring these lesions. Nonetheless, series of patients with *both* MCD *and* reflex seizures are not found in the literature. This may be due either to underreporting or, alternatively, to unknown specific mechanisms rendering patients with MCD relatively resistant to reflex seizures, in spite of their cortical hyperexcitability.

The present chapter describes nine patients with MCD and reflex seizures, recruited from seven different epilepsy centres, which is in itself an indication that this is a rare association. The discussion that follows the case reports below will address both the mechanisms through which reflex seizures could occur in patients with MCD, and also speculative insights on why these seizures are (paradoxically) rare in these patients.

Case reports

Patient #1, S.Y.

This 5-year-old girl was born at term from nonconsanguineous parents, following an uneventful pregnancy and delivery. Epileptic spasms began at four months of age, and a neurogenetic evaluation showed a deletion at the large arm of chromosome 11 (46, XX, del (11)(q22.2q23.2)), which contains a NCAM gene (*Figure 1a*). Both parents have normal karyotypes. Physical examination, including an ophthalmologic evaluation, showed only low implantation of both ears, being otherwise unremarkable. Screening for inborn errors of metabolism was negative, but a 1.5 T MRI revealed abnormal gyration in both parieto-occipital regions, more marked on the right (*Figure 1b*). She evolved with mental retardation (developmental quotient = 50). Initial interictal EEGs showed a generalised hypsarrhythmic pattern. After several months, however, she began with partial seizures with clinical and EEG features

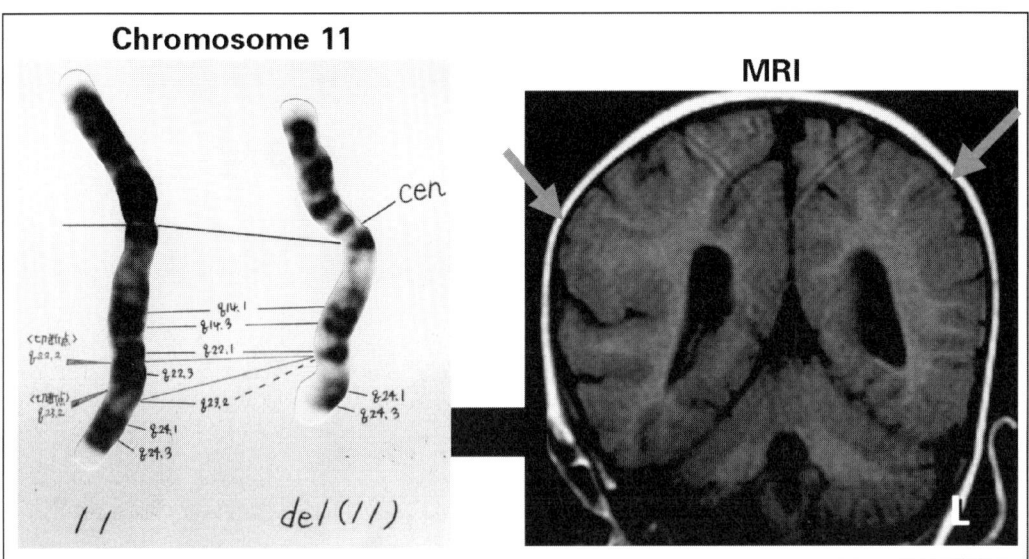

Figure 1. Chromosome analysis (a) and coronal T1-weighted MRI section (b) showing deletion at the large arm of chromosome 11 (46, XX, del (11)(q22.2q23.2)) and a cortical malformation (increased thickness and abnormal gyration) in the posterior quadrants, predominating in the right.

suggestive of frontal lobe onset, which were controlled by zonisamide. Around age two she started with self-induced reflex seizures characterized by brief tonic posturing, triggered by forced eye deviation to left combined with forced blinking. These were resistant to zonisamide, but were eventually controlled by dexamethasone. She never had photoparoxysmal EEG responses.

Patient #2, A.V.

This boy was evaluated at age seven years. He was the product of an uneventful pregnancy and delivery, walked at 30 months and began saying a few words at 36 months. Seizures started when he was three, characterized by clonic and then dystonic movements of the left hemibody, eventually involving all four limbs. At around the same age, startle-induced tonic drop attacks began, ushered in by unexpected sound or touch. If he was distracted and someone patted his back he would fall, recovering immediately. The family needed to adapt to his seizures in several ways, and telephone and door rings had to be disconnected. They also had to move from their house close to the city airport, since the patient would have several drop attacks a day during airplane landing and take off. He was hyperactive, disinhibited, and had frequent episodes of temper tantrums. Behaviour abnormalities and frequent seizure recurrence made school attendance impossible. He had a mild left hemiparesis and an ataxic gait. Genetic evaluation was normal. Interictal EEGs showed diffuse slowing of background activity, multifocal spikes, and secondary bilateral synchrony. Drop attacks were accompanied by irregular, brief, generalised spike-wave complexes.

MRI showed diffuse band heterotopia, with minimal abnormalities of the overlying cortex (*Figure 2*). He failed several antiepileptic drug regimens as well as a complete callosotomy, and eventually died of status epilepticus at age 14.

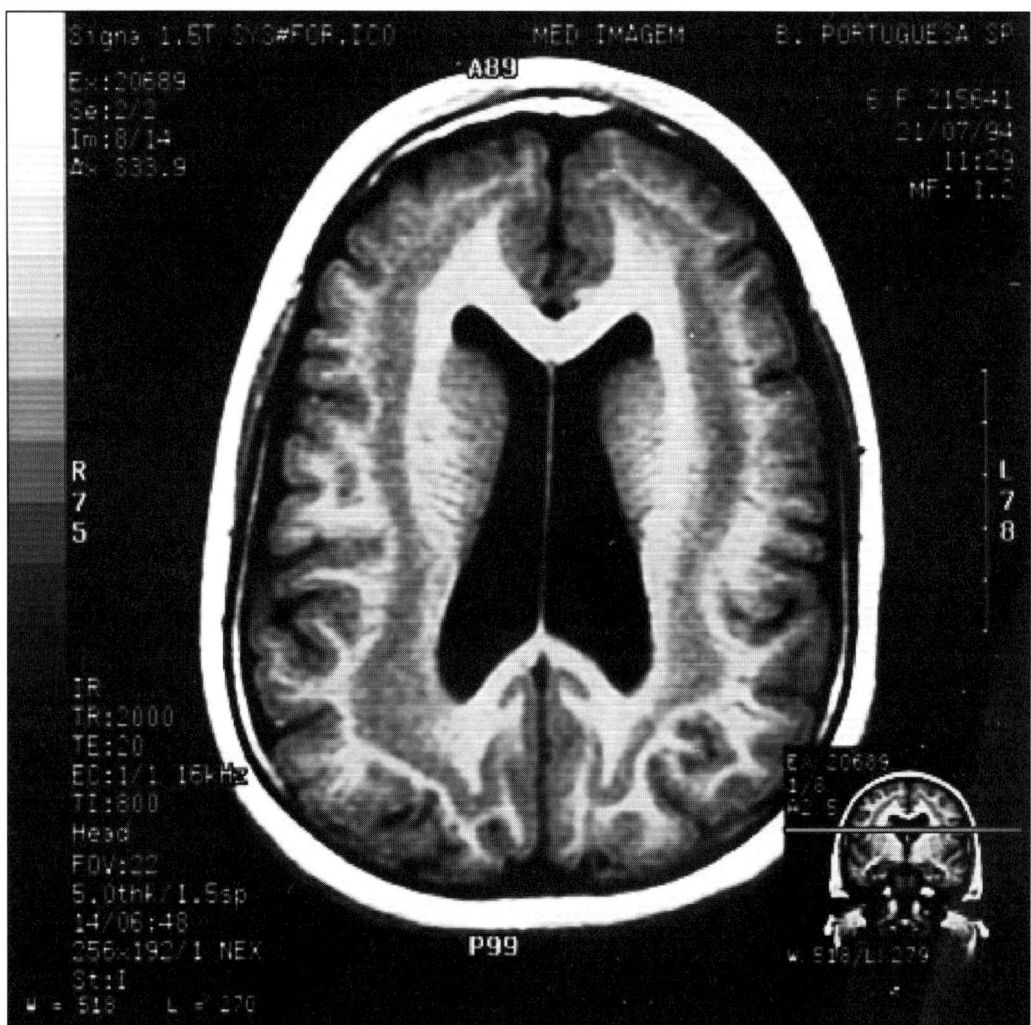

Figure 2. Axial T1-weighted MRI section shows diffuse bilateral subcortical band heterotopia.

Patient #3, A.A.

This 27-year-old woman was the product of uneventful pregnancy and delivery, but had difficulties sucking and swallowing since birth. She sat at 12 and walked at 18 months. Word comprehension was noted from 18 months, but the first few words were uttered only at age four. Speech developed in the context of severe dysarthria and limitation of tongue movements. Seizures started at age 11, and manifested in different ways. Most commonly, she has staring episodes with minimal perioral movements which occasionally progressed to secondarily generalised tonic-clonic seizures.

She also has drop attacks and, in addition, there are frequent episodes of perioral myoclonia, induced by eating or talking over the phone. In many of these episodes there is a stereotyped sequence: while eating or talking over the phone she stares, has perioral myoclonia, and falls backwards. Neurologic examination shows mild diffuse spasticity, and severe pseudobulbar signs. She is overtly dysarthric, and cannot protrude or move the tongue laterally. There is constant salivation. Interictal EEGs show bilateral centrotemporal spikes, occasionally associated with diffuse, generalised irregular spike and wave complexes. Ictal EEG shows bilateral rhythmic activity, with frontocentrotemporal predominance. MRI displays bilateral, roughly symmetrical, perisylvian polymicrogyria. Seizures were not controlled with different combinations of antiepileptic drugs, and she also failed anterior callosotomy.

Patient #4, A.S.

This 51-year-old man has reflex seizures associated with an imaging abnormality suggestive of focal cortical dysplasia in the left centro-insular region. He has mild cognitive impairment and a FSIQ of 82. Pregnancy and delivery were normal. Seizures started at age three, and may take different forms of presentation. Some are characterized by brief, dystonic contractions of both arms followed by complex pedalling automatisms. During wakefulness these episodes are preceded by an aura of "impending catastrophe". Alternatively, he has clonic movements of the right face, arm and leg. In addition, he has seizures precipitated by meals or "gastric fullness". These may present only as perioral myoclonia associated with head turning to the right, or progress into a secondary generalised seizure. Neurologic examination is unremarkable. Interictal and ictal EEGs do not display epileptogenic abnormalities. MRI shows an area of blurring of the grey-white matter transition and increased fluid-attenuation inversion recovery signal in the left inferior central and insular region *(Figure 3)*. Seizures have been refractory to different antiepileptic drug combinations in high dosages. He is currently being considered for surgical treatment.

Patient #5, C.D.M.

This 15-year-old right-handed girl is the only child of nonconsanguineous parents. Her mother had previously had two spontaneous abortions, and her pregnancy was complicated by bleeding in the first trimester. Delivery was through cesarean section, with mild perinatal distress. She developed normally, without feeding difficulties, and attends a regular school. Family history is negative for epilepsy, but both her grandmother and her only aunt have mild dysarthria. Seizures started with sudden, brief episodes of grunting and sialorrhea during sleep at age six. These were controlled with carbamazepine, but resumed at age nine, in the form of brief disconnection from the surroundings followed by head dropping. Vigabatrin controlled these attacks for three additional years, when at age 12 medically refractory seizures ensued. These occur many times a day, either as episodes characterized by sudden vocalization (a "grunt", a "hiccup" or an "eructation") followed by myoclonus of the head and upper extremities – to the point that objects may fall from her hands – or as more prolonged attacks beginning with head turning to the right and followed by staring and dystonic posturing of the right extremities. Following this latter type of seizures, speech

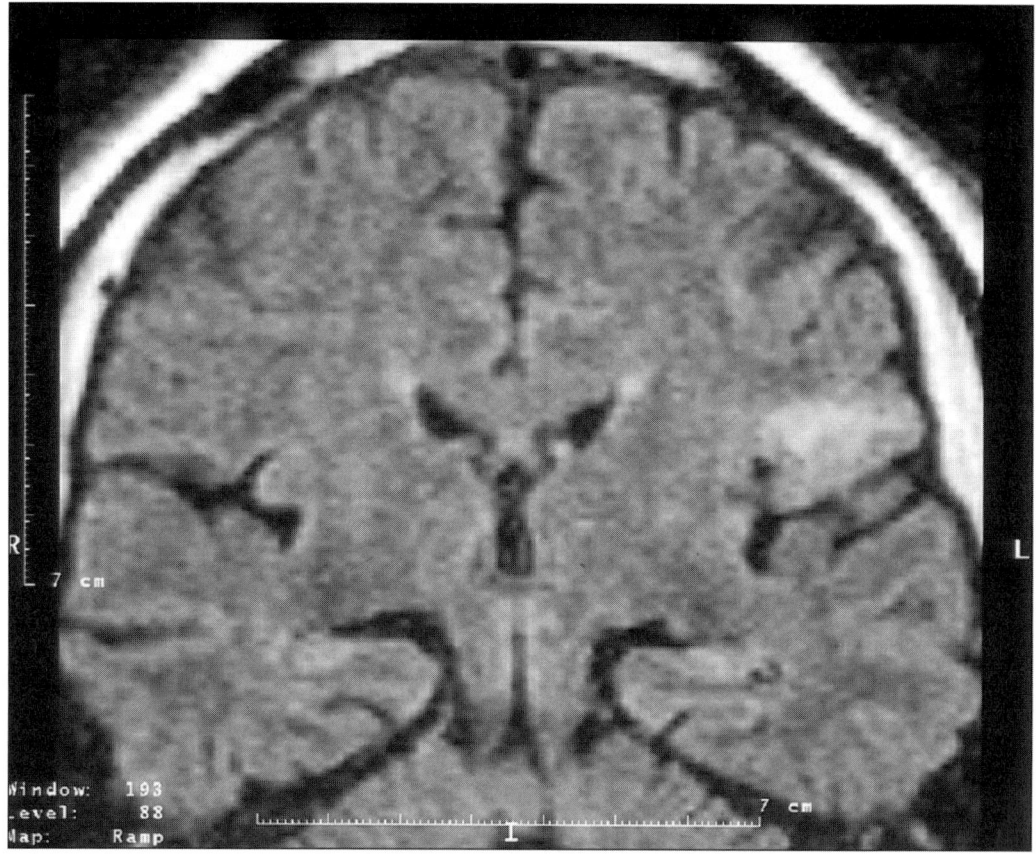

Figure 3. Coronal MRI section acquired with fluid-attenuated inversion recovery (FLAIR) showing increased cortico-subcortical signal in the left centro-insular region.

becomes transiently dysarthric. Seizures tend to cluster around meals, either while she is actually eating, about to eat, or talking about eating. For instance, during video-EEG monitoring she had one seizure while facing the food tray and another while discussing the food placed in front of her. In several different occasions, however, no seizures were provoked by drinking orange juice. Neurological examination shows mild orolingual dyspraxia. She can protrude and move the tongue from side to side, but cannot produce clicking sounds or perform other complex lingual movements. Moreover, she cannot whistle or inflate a balloon. Dysarthria, however, is only minimal and intelligence is normal. EEGs show bilateral centrotemporal discharges, predominating in the left midtemporal region *(Figure 4)*. Ictal episodes are accompanied by diffuse EEG changes, with a maximum over the left temporal region. MRI shows bilateral frontal, parietal, and perisylvian polymicrogyria, more severe on the left side, where the insula is fully exposed through an open operculum *(Figure 5)*. Functional MRI shows that the polymicrogyric cortex has retained motor function bilaterally, and language functions are lateralised to the left hemisphere.

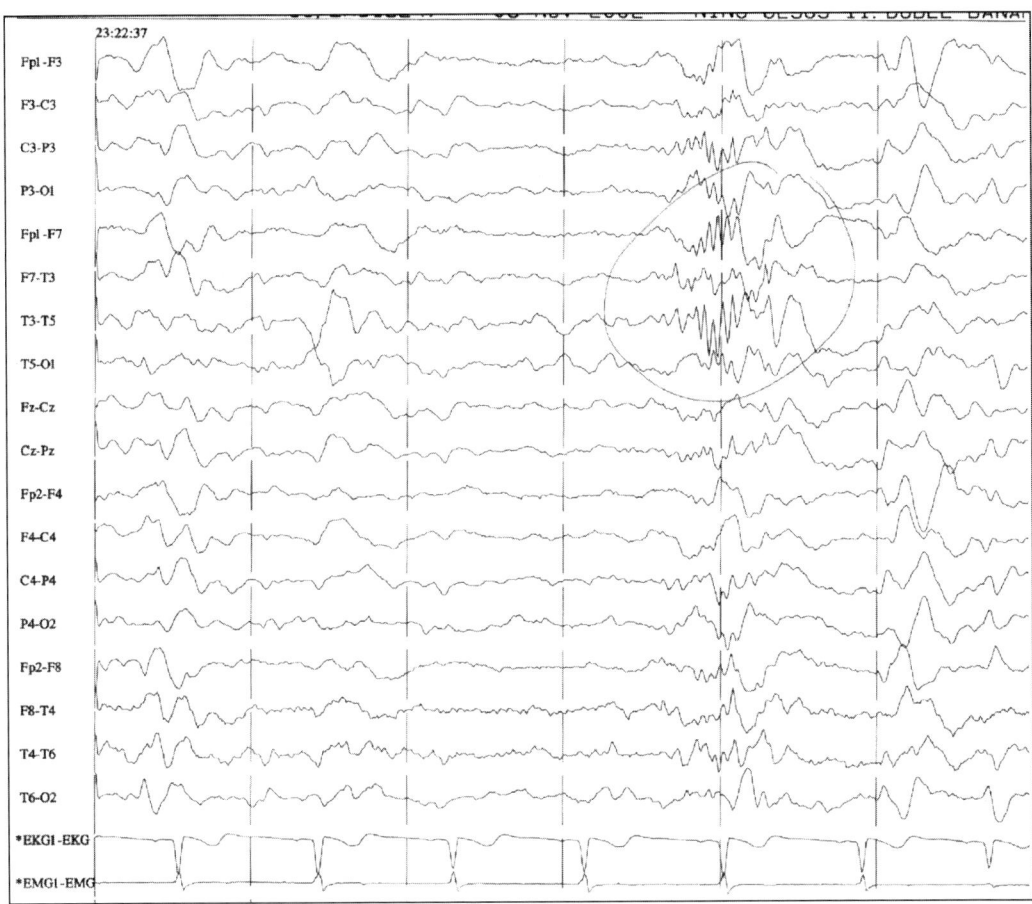

Figure 4. Interictal EEG showing epileptiform discharges in the centro-temporal regions bilaterally, predominating on the left.

Patient #6 L.C.A.

This 14-year-old boy was initially seen at age seven for medically refractory seizures, which started at age three. At evaluation he had several attacks a week, in which the left arm and leg would become dystonic and he would fall if standing. In addition, he had sudden drop attacks if a loud sound or a stroke on his back would come unattended. He was attending special school and had a history of delayed acquisition of developmental milestone, having walked only around two years of age. There was no history of significant perinatal distress. Neurological examination showed diffuse hypotonia. Interictal EEGs showed trains of spikes involving the right anterior quadrant and frequent diffuse paroxysmal discharges suggestive of secondary bilateral synchrony. Production of a sudden loud noise during a video-EEG recording led to global myoclonus and an irregular burst of diffuse spike and wave complexes. MRI (0.5T) showed blurring of the grey-white matter transition diffusely in the right frontal lobe. During operation, ECoG showed continuous sharp waves over the right

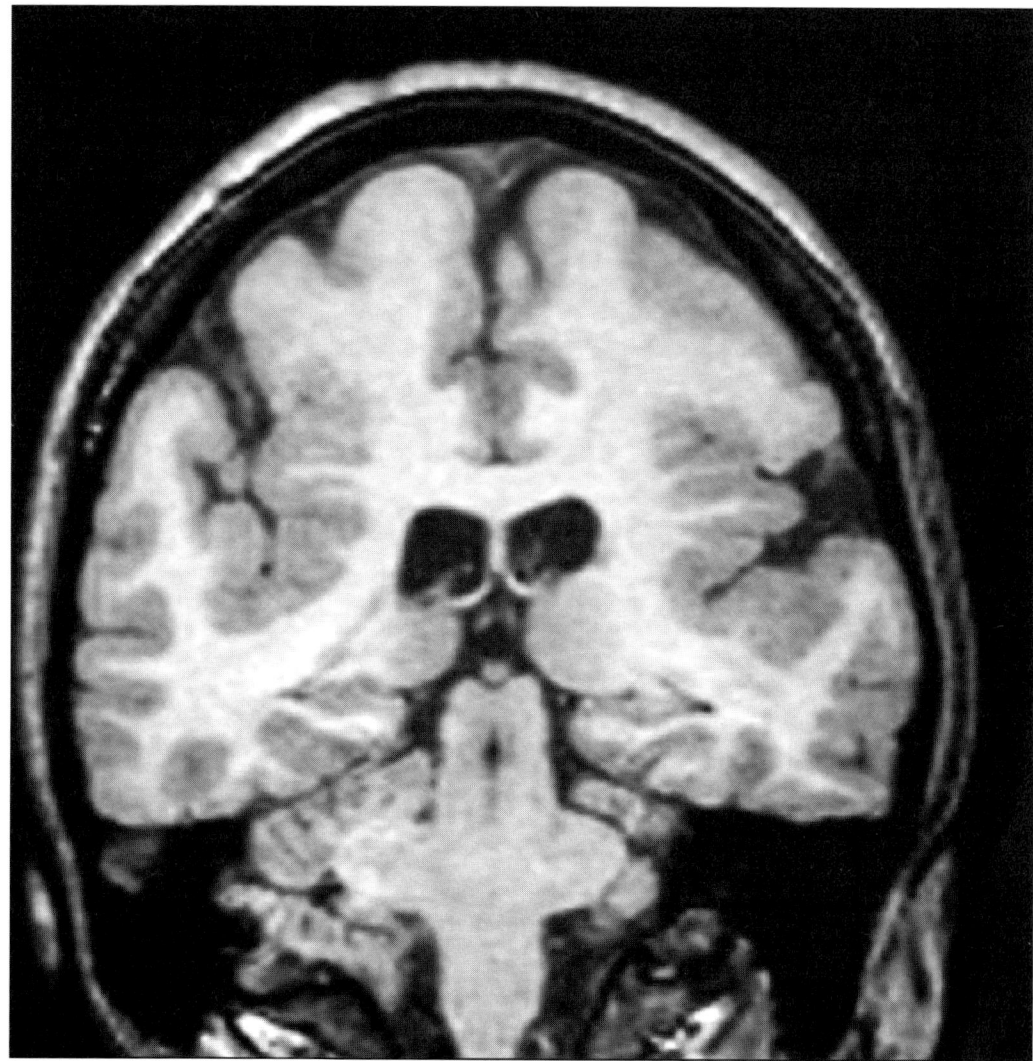

Figure 5. Coronal T1-weighted MRI shows bilateral perisylvian polymicrogyria.

frontal lobe, which was largely resected. A histological pattern characteristic of Taylor-type focal cortical dysplasia, with dysplastic neurons and balloon cells was identified in the resected tissue. The patient was seizure-free for five years, and then had recurrence of some simple partial motor seizures involving the left arm. He has had no further falls, even when startled.

Patient #7, O.R.

A 17-year-old right-handed woman presented with a three-year history of spontaneously occurring tonic-clonic seizures of the right thumb and index finger. She had also noticed that these occurred and could be elicited voluntarily when she rubbed salt, sugar, sand, bread crumbs or silk between her right thumb and index finger. A single nocturnal secondarily generalised tonic-clonic seizure was also reported. Two seizures could be evoked during video-EEG monitoring using sugar. The initial unpleasant tonic posturing of the hand and forearm was followed by a 2-4 Hz clonus of the thumb, accompanied by an EEG seizure pattern, regional left frontoparietal, maximum at C3 (*Figure 6*). Postictal testing revealed a sensory deficit of the whole right thumb and the tip of the index finger. Sensory stimulation alone or finger movements without sugar, salt, etc. were insufficient to evoke seizures. The MRI was normal. Median nerve SSEP were normal except for a decreased amplitude of the later components following P25. The P37 amplitude was higher after right-sided stimulation. Seizure frequency was reduced by carbamazepine. Considering the nonlesional MRI, focal cortical dysplasia was felt to be the most likely aetiology, even though there is no firm evidence for this hypothesis.

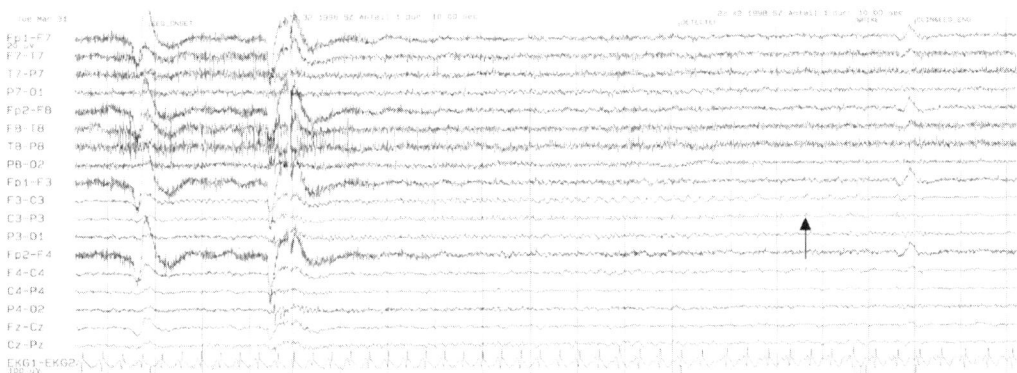

Figure 6. The EEG-seizure pattern, regional left central is shown. The small spikes visible at C3 (arrow) occurred time-locked with the twitches of the right thumb.

Patients #8 and #9

These two patients are described in detail elsewhere (Palmini *et al.*, submitted). In brief, patient 8 is a 15-year-old boy with episodes in which the he stares at a white paper or a shiny surface, and then has a tonic seizure with stiffening of the upper limbs and loss of awareness for about 10 seconds. These always occur on awakening as he tries persistently to evoke a seizure, since he "feels good when he has a stare". What he means is that he feels warm and fuzzy after these episodes, and has been instructed to at least sit down before provoking the episodes to prevent injuries. Unfortunately, in several occasions he has suffered severe injuries due to drop attacks. MRI demonstrates severe cerebellar hypoplasia and extensive subependymal heterotopia on both sides, extending into the temporal horns from the posterior horns. In addition, there is severe right mesial occipital dysplasia, with extensive patchy hyperintensity in the white matter posteriorly on both sides. Patient 9 is a 34-year-old woman of normal intelligence, which has seizures induced by rubbing the sole of the right foot or by urinary bladder distension. Neurophysiologic evaluation confirmed an epileptogenic zone in the left primary somatosensory cortex in the mesial aspect of the frontoparietal regions, which was shown to be related to a Taylor-type focal cortical dysplasia [13].

Discussion

Mechanisms leading to reflex seizures

Reflex seizures represent hyperexcitable responses of intracortical circuits to specific afferent stimuli. The cerebral cortex is constantly bombarded with afferent exteroceptive and interoceptive sensory information, and whichever the nature of the stimulus *at least* two types of sensorimotor loops are constantly being activated, one short, and one long (multisynaptic). The short loops bypass the more refined processing of the sensory stimulus and tend to lead to some kind of reflex motor response. Long intracortical loops, on the other hand, extend through sequential "stations" of processing of the afferent stimulus, and lead to nonreflex, goal-directed motor responses. A number of cortical and subcortical structures regulate the activation of sensorimotor loops, thus modulating response to stimuli according to the specific contingencies of the moment [15-17]. It can be hypothesized that reflex seizures derive from pathological hyperexcitability of short sensorimotor loops, which lead not only to uninhibited reflex motor responses, but actually to *sustained, excessive motor responses to specific stimuli*.

One puzzling issue is why even within the background of diffuse regional hyperexcitability of sensorimotor networks thought to be associated with dysplastic lesions, only a very specific stimulus in a given modality gives rise to reflex seizures. Why is it that in patient 1 only fixed staring (and not other types of visual stimuli), or in patient 2 only left-sided gaze and blinking, activate hyperexcitable loops? It is possible that despite overall hyperexcitability there are still several levels of inhibition which are overcome only through specific "neural channels", activated by very specific types of stimuli. Irrespective of the mechanisms involved, electrophysiological studies including EEG, evoked potentials, and back-averaging of reflex motor responses suggest that sensorimotor loops are indeed hyperexcitable in patients with reflex seizures [15-18]. MCD would be, at least theoretically, compatible with such levels of hyperexcitability.

Mechanisms of hyperexcitability in MCD

The mechanisms associated with intrinsic and enhanced epileptogenicity in MCD have been studied through different techniques, which examined the morphologic, physiologic, and neurochemical characteristics of the dysplastic tissue. Morphological studies point to persistent "epileptogenic" plasticity and abnormal connectivity in different forms of MCD. For instance, it has been suggested that large dysplastic neurons and balloon cells (fingerprints of the Taylor-type of FCD) may escape programmed cell death through continuous expression of neurotrophins and *trk* receptor proteins, thus modelling and augmenting their synaptic network through retained active neurite plasticity [19]. In addition, it has been demonstrated that immature neurons in heterotopic positions can make reciprocal connections with the neocortex and with other heterotopic aggregates, probably creating networks of hyperexcitability.

Robust neurophysiologic evidence for intrinsic epileptogenicity was recently obtained in *in vitro* studies of slices of brain tissue resected from patients with medically refractory focal cortical dysplasia maintained *in vitro*. In the presence of 4-aminopyridine, a K+ channel blocker which increases transmitter release, spontaneous, prolonged epileptiform discharges resembling electrographic seizures were recorded from these slices. The dependence of this activity on excitatory amino acid receptors was demonstrated by its disappearance upon the application of NMDA (N-methyl-D-aspartate) and AMPA (d-amino-3-hydroxy-5-methyl-4-isoxazolepropionic acid) receptor antagonists [20]. Immunocytochemical studies are also shedding light on the biological counterparts of the increased and intrinsic epileptogenicity of focal cortical dysplasia. These studies have consistently shown a decreased density of inhibitory GABAergic interneurons and an increase in the number of abnormally oriented pyramidal cells displaying positive immunostaining for excitatory amino acid receptors (Spreafico, 1998 #80; Spreafico, 2000 #81; Ying, 2002 #82).

Clinical and neurophysiological counterparts of increased epileptogenicity in MCD

Clinical and neurophysiological evidence also support the contention that MCD are highly epileptogenic and thus prone to be associated with reflex seizures. The intrinsic epileptogenicity of these lesions is further supported by their frequent association with epilepsia partialis continua and other types of status epilepticus (Andermann, 1992 #73; Costa da Costa, 1996 #37; Desbiens, 1993 #74; Kuzniecky, 1993 #75; Palmini, 1991 #76; Silva, 1995 #77). In addition, these lesions often produce continuous epileptogenic discharges recorded on the scalp EEG or directly over the lesion on ECoG [5-7, 21]. Taken in conjunction with the well-known anatomical predisposition of these lesions to be localised around or extend to perirolandic sensorimotor cortex [1, 22, 23], these features suggest that epileptogenic loops in sensorimotor and other regions are poorly inhibited, with a resulting net hyperexcitability.

Putative mechanisms of reflex seizures in MCD

In view of the data discussed above, it is understandable that the patients reported here had reflex seizures as part of their epilepsies. It is likely that there are different mechanisms of increased epileptogenicity modulating the different forms of MCD represented in our patients [12]. Some may be related to the presence of grossly abnormal cells and to modified intracortical circuitry, as is the case of patients 4, 7, and 9 who have confirmed or probable Taylor-type focal cortical dysplasia. The mechanisms underlying the epileptogenicity of polymicrogyria are not clear, although experimental models of this malformation are consistently associated with seizures. Polymicrogyric cortex, as seen in patients 3 and 5, probably has not only abnormal connectivity with surrounding tissue but the redundant gyri probably also lead to an anatomical propensity for short circuit loops, one of the prerequisites for the generation of reflex seizures [24, 25]. Patients with subcortical heterotopia probably derive their hyperexcitability from aberrant connectivity between subcortically placed and cortical neurons [26-28]. This has been recently demonstrated both for nodular subcortical as well as for band heterotopia, and could be reasonable explanations for reflex seizures in patients 1, 2, and 8. Irrespective of the intrinsic mechanisms, however, MCD would appear to be in a favourable position to generate reflex seizures.

Why reflex seizures are rare in patients with MCD – A hypothesis

In spite of the enhanced epileptogenic features of MCD, reflex seizures are infrequent in patients with these disorders. In a consecutive series of 154 patients studied in Porto Alegre and Montreal, only five of 164 patients (3%) had reflex seizures: two of 112 with FCD, two of 28 with bilateral perisylvian polymicrogyria, and one of 24 with subcortical band heterotopia had reflex seizures (Palmini et al., unpublished observations). Previously reported patients from this series include a 15-year-old boy with a right parieto-occipital FCD and seizures induced by drinking or eating [29] and a recently reported man with temporal lobe complex partial seizures consistently induced by thinking about his father looking at him at his childhood home. MRI and pathology showed a Taylor-type focal cortical dysplastic lesion in the left anterior temporal lobe [30]. Reviewing the literature spanning the MRI era, only a few more patients are reported in whom reflex seizures had a MCD as the underlying aetiology [31].

These low figures raise the issue of why reflex seizures are uncommon in patients with MCD. One possibility is that clinical history in patients known to have MCDs is not addressing features related to reflex seizure. However, this is not the most likely explanation, since most patients with reflex seizures spontaneously identify and report specific seizure precipitants and often seek an adequate explanation for the relationship between the specific stimulus and the seizures. Another possibility is that MCDs, while being intrinsically epileptogenic, have poorly developed extralesional connectivity, and do not form functional recurrent excitation loops with surrounding cortical and subcortical structures. This could amount to a "natural protection" against reflex seizures. However, this possibility is not supported by functional anatomic data showing that heterotopic neurons do form strong connections with other brain regions [27, 28]. Another possibility is that MCD, while displaying increased levels of epileptogenicity, might also be associated with distributed inhibitory networks. Several patients with MCD undergoing epilepsy surgery have been shown to present postoperative seizures starting days to months following lesion resection, and originating from previously unsuspected epileptogenic regions, at a distance or even contralateral to the site of resection [32-34]. It is reasonable to assume that these "secondary epileptogenic regions" were under inhibitory influence of the primary lesion, and only manifested clinically after resection of the latter. Thus, the paucity of reports of reflex seizures in patients with MCD should stimulate research on the relationship between inhibitory and excitatory influences in these malformed brains.

References

1. Palmini A. Disorders of cortical development. *Curr Opin Neurol* 2000; 13: 183-92.
2. Semah F, Picot MC, Adam MD, et al. Is the underlying cause of epilepsy a major prognostic factor for recurrence? *Neurology* 1998; 51: 1256-62.
3. Tassi L, Colombo N, Garbelli R, et al. Focal cortical dysplasia: neuropathological subtypes, EEG, neuroimaging and surgical outcome. *Brain* 2002; 125: 1719-32.
4. Costa da Costa J, Palmini A, Andermann F, et al. Epilepsia Vs, 1996. Epilepsia partialis continua associated with rolandic cortical dysplasia: Delineation of a specific subsyndrome. *Epilepsia* 1996; 37 (suppl. 5): 37.
5. Dubeau F, Palmini A, Fish D, et al. The significance of electrocorticographic findings in focal cortical dysplasia: a review of their clinical, electrophysiological and neurochemical characteristics. *Electroencephalogr Clin Neurophysiol* 1998; 48 (suppl.): 77-96.
6. Gambardella A, Palmini A, Andermann F, et al. Usefulness of focal rhythmic discharges on scalp EEG of patients with focal cortical dysplasia and intractable epilepsy. *EEG Clin Neurophysiol* 1996; 98: 243-9.
7. Palmini A, Gambardella A, Andermann F, et al. Intrinsic epileptogenicity of human dysplastic cortex as suggested by corticography and surgical results. *Ann Neurol* 1995; 37: 476-87.
8. Babb TL, Ying Z, Hadam J, Penrod C. Glutamate receptor mechanisms in human epileptic dysplastic cortex. *Epilepsy Res* 1998; 32: 24-33.
9. Ferrer I, Pineda M, Tallada M. Abnormal local circuit neurons in epilepsia partialis continua associated with focal cortical dysplasia. *Acta Neuropathol* (Berl) 1992; 83: 647-52.
10. Spreafico R, Tassi L, Colombo N, et al. Inhibitory circuits in human dysplastic tissue. *Epilepsia* 2000; 41 (suppl. 6): S168-73.
11. Ying Z, Najm I. Mechanisms of epileptogenicity in focal malformations caused by abnormal cortical development. *Neurosurg Clin North Am* 2002; 13: 27-24.
12. Palmini A, da Costa JC, Calcagnotto ME, Paglioli-Neto E, Paglioli E, Coutinho L. Patients with specific histopathological types of cortical dysplasia have specific degrees of severity of the epileptic condition. A study of 78 patients. *Epilepsia* 1997; 38 (suppl. 3): 5.
13. Palmini A, Lüders HO. Classification issues in malformations caused by abnormalities of cortical development. *Neurosurg Clin North Am* 2002; 13: 1-16.
14. Biraben A, Scarabin JM, de Toffol B, Vignal JP, Chauvel PY. Opercular reflex seizures: a case report with stereoelectroencephalographic demonstration. *Epilepsia* 1999; 40: 655-63.
15. Naquet RG, Valin A. Experimental models of reflex epilepsy. *Adv Neurol* 1998; 75: 15-27.
16. Wieser HG. Seizure induction in reflex seizures and reflex epilepsies. *Adv Neurol* 1998; 75: 69-85.
17. Wolf P, Goosses R. Relationship of photosensitivity to epileptic syndromes. *J Neurol Neurosurg Psychiatry* 1986; 49: 1386-91.
18. Kasteleijn-Nolst Trenité D. Photosensitivity in epilepsy: electrophysiological and clinical correlates. *Acta Neurol Scand* 1989; 80 (suppl. 125): 1-149.
19. Nishio S, Morioka T, Hamada Y, Hisada K, Fukui M. Immunohistochemical expression of trk receptor proteins in focal cortical dysplasia with intractable epilepsy. *Neuropathol Appl Neurobiol* 1999; 25: 188-95.
20. Avoli M, Bernasconi A, Mattia D, Olivier A, Hwa GGC. Epileptiform discharges in the human dysplastic neocortex: *in vitro* physiology and pharmacology. *Ann Neurol* 1999; 46: 816-26.
21. Rosenow F, Lüders HO, Dinner DS, et al. Histopathological correlates of epileptogenicity as expressed by electrocorticographic spiking and seizure frequency. *Epilepsia* 1998; 39: 850-6.
22. Andermann F. Epilepsia partialis continua and other seizures arising from the precentral gyrus: high incidence in patients with Rasmussen's syndrome and neuronal migration disorders. *Brain Dev* 1992; 14: 338-9.

23. Kuzniecky R, Morawetz R, Faught E, Black L. Frontal and central lobe focal dysplasia: clinical, EEG and imaging features. *Dev Med Child Neurol* 1995; 37: 159-66.
24. Dvorak K, Feit J, Jurankova Z. Experimentally induced focal microgyria and status verrucosis deformis in rats: pathogenesis and interrelation, histological and autoradiographical study. *Acta Neuropathol* (Berl) 1978; 44: 121-9.
25. Hablitz JJ, DeFazio T. Excitability changes in freeze-induced neocortical microgyria. *Epilepsy Res* 1998; 32: 75-82.
26. Chevassus-au-Louis N, Represa A. The right neuron at the wrong place: biology of heterotopic neurons in cortical neuronal migration disorders, with special reference to associated pathologies. *Cell Mol Life Sci* 1999; 55: 1206-15.
27. Colacitti C, Sancini G, Franceschetti S, *et al*. Altered connections between neocortical and heterotopic areas in methylazoxymethanol-treated rat. *Epilepsy Res* 1998; 32: 49-62.
28. Hannan AJ, Servotte S, Kastnelson A, *et al*. Characterization of nodular neuronal heterotopia in children. *Brain* 1999; 122: 219-38.
29. Verdu A, Ruiz-Falco ML. Eating seizures associated with focal cortical dysplasia. *Brain Dev* 1991; 13: 352-4.
30. Martinez O, Reisin R, Andermann F, Zifkin BG, Sevlever G. Evidence for reflex activation of experiential complex partial seizures. *Neurology* 2001; 56: 121-3.
31. Manford MR, Fish DR, Shorvon SD. Startle provoked epileptic seizures: features in 19 patients. *J Neurol Neurosurg Psychiatry* 1996; 61: 151-6.
32. Molyneux PD, Barker RA, Thom M, Van Paesschen W, Harkness WF, Duncan JS. Successful treatment of epilepsia partialis continua with multiple subpial transections. *J Neurol Neurosurg Psychiatry* 1997: 137-8.
33. Palmini A, da Costa JC, Calcagnotto ME, Oliveira AJ, Paglioli-Neto E, Paglioli E. Unexpected, unwelcome surprises after surgical excision of apparently localised cortical dysplastic lesions: "de novo" clinical and electrographical manifestations of unsuspected, imaging-negative, remote lesions. *Epilepsia* 1997; 38 (suppl. 3): 31-3.
34. Sisodiya SM. Surgery for malformations of cortical development causing epilepsy. *Brain* 2000; 123: 1075-91.

In the same collection
current problems in epilepsy series

J. Roger : *Epileptic Syndromes in Infancy, Childhood and Adolescence* (3rd edition). Paris : Ed John Libbey Eurotext, 2002, vol. 18, 544 pages.

C.P. Panayiotopoulos : *Panayiotopoulos Syndrome : A Common and Benign Childhood Epileptic Syndrome.* Paris : Ed John Libbey Eurotext, 2002, vol. 17, 120 pages.

M. Pfäfflin : *Comprehensive Care for People with Epilepsy.* Paris : Ed John Libbey Eurotext, vol. 16, 2001, 372 pages.

C.P. Panayiotopoulos : *Benign Childhood Partial Seizures and Related Epileptic Syndromes.* Paris : Ed John Libbey Eurotext, 1999, vol 15, 416 pages.

A. Nehlig : Childhood Epilepsies and Brain development. Paris : Ed John Libbey Eurotext, 1999, vol. 14, 320 pages.

S.F. Berkovic : *Genetics of Focal Epilepsies.* Paris : Ed John Libbey Eurotext, 1999, vol. 13, 296 pages.

G. Avanzini : *Molecular and Cellular Targets for Anti-Epileptic Drugs.* Paris : Ed John Libbey Eurotext, 1997, vol. 12, 272 pages.

I. Tuxhorn : *Paediatric Epilepsy Syndromes and Their Surgical Treatment.* Paris : Ed John Libbey Eurotext, 1997, vol. 11, 894 pages.

P. Wolf : *Epileptic Seizures and Syndromes.* Paris : Ed John Libbey Eurotext, 1994, vol. 10, 688 pages.

Achevé d'imprimer par Corlet, Imprimeur, S.A.
14110 Condé-sur-Noireau
N° d'Imprimeur : 79637 - Dépôt légal : novembre 2004

Imprimé en France